Low Intensity Laser Therapy in Clinical Practice

Fred Kahn, MD, FRCS(C)

Published 2006-04-20

Meditech International Inc.
411 Horner Ave, Unit #1
Toronto, ON
Canada
M8W 4W3

Tel: (416) 251 1055
Fax: (416) 251 2446
e-mail: info@bioflexlaser.com
web site: www.bioflexlaser.com

The author gratefully acknowledges the invaluable contribution of Leslie Perrin and Michael Patterson in the preparation of this manuscript.

Contact Meditech International Inc. for clarification and further information regarding the protocols prescribed in this document.

Disclaimer: Meditech International Inc. adheres to recommended safety standards and proven treatment outcome methodologies. The company has a comprehensive training program that health care professionals using the BioFlex Professional System, should follow, in order to properly conduct treatment strategies in applying LILT. Meditech International does not support the incorrect application of LILT.

Printed by DIBO Canada Inc.
Printed in Canada

Foreword

Low intensity laser therapy (LILT) has been used for over 30 years to treat a wide range of clinical conditions including acute and chronic musculoskeletal disorders, rheumatoid arthritis peripheral arterial occlusive disease, chronic wounds and osteoarthritis. Success depends on accurate diagnosis and appropriate application of LILT. In a series of essays and treatment protocols, Dr. Fred Kahn, describes the philosophy underlying his use of LILT in the treatment of these disorders and explains how success can be achieved. In addition to being an expert in the clinical application of LILT and an entrepreneur, Dr. Kahn is also a surgeon. Refreshingly, he is a surgeon who believes that for many conditions, surgery should be the last resort. He has found, over some 16 years during which he and his colleagues have treated approximately 100,000 patients with LILT, that in these patients this last resort is rarely required. In this book he shares with us his unique experience, acquired from the treatment of these patients.

Although primarily for clinicians, this book will also be of great value to those investigating the mechanisms by which LILT produces its effects. Knowledge of what can be achieved clinically when LILT is applied appropriately will inform future research. The book is an excellent training manual and reference book for clinicians using LILT. Protocols for using the BioFlex Professional System, developed by Dr. Kahn, are clearly described and illustrated.

I am certain that all who read this book, whatever their current level of knowledge of LILT or their clinical expertise, will learn much from it. Most importantly, patients will benefit as more clinicians acquire the skills necessary to apply LILT successfully.

I have no hesitation in recommending this excellent book to present and future users of LILT. It will have pride of place in my library and be referred to frequently.

M. Dyson

Mary Dyson, Ph.D., C. Biol., F.A.I.U.M. (Hon)

Introduction

What began as a tentative exploration of the world of Low Intensity Laser Therapy in 1988 is emerging as an international enterprise of considerable proportion. During the past year, Meditech certified over two hundred Laser Therapists at its corporate facility. Over the next year, we expect to educate and train over five hundred more. These include physicians, chiropractors, physiotherapists and other related medical disciplines. Initially, the courses were based on a monthly schedule, but due to overwhelming demand are now held on an almost weekly basis.

Our products are established in twenty two countries including hospital based physiotherapy facilities, physiatry centers, major university health institutions and a chiropractic school in addition to a growing number of professional sports franchises. We have become the world leaders in shifting from the concept of pain management to the reality of curing many complex disease entities. Our significant improvement/cure rate continues to be in excess of the 90% range.

Whereas with acute problems and in the younger age groups total resolution of problems is readily achieved. In the older age groups suffering from chronic degenerative processes, regeneration of cells along with the concomitant elimination of symptoms, results in the continuing improvement of treatment outcomes. Surgical solutions such as joint replacement and decompression procedures for stenosis of the spinal canal are rapidly being replaced by Low Intensity Laser Therapy along with the elimination of analgesics and other pharmaceuticals. This allows patients to resume normal activities and return to work, a process that has now become the standard.

Through "word of mouth" communications, the influx of patients continues to flow to our clinics from points such as Paris, Geneva, New York, etc. on an ongoing basis. Frequently, patients are so impressed with the result of the treatment that they bring in their personal physicians to be similarly helped, albeit grudgingly on occasion. Unfortunately, many years of conditioning in the medical sector has created a focus based on prescriptions, lab studies and cross-consultation without inroads on therapeutic progress. At Meditech, we set an example by treating the clinical problem in a direct, simple and effective manner. With our approach almost invariably the pathology is resolved in rapid fashion. Following the clinical assessment, treatment is initiated and as I always tell patients "the sooner you begin treatment, the sooner you will become well."

Next year, we plan to introduce new products to the marketplace in our endeavor to maintain the standard of continuing excellence. The staff at Meditech continues to grow and with the inclusion of our manufacturing facility now numbers over forty individuals. It has become company policy to retain more postgraduate university students along with a selective number of outside consultants to enable our efforts to become more focused and efficient. In addition to our clinics where over 1000 patient treatments are rendered on a weekly basis, we are establishing a strong educational facility that promotes the understanding and application of laser therapy.

The learning curve is less intimidating than it was sixteen years ago; however, many challenges remain and are systematically being overcome. We are grateful for the assistance in our endeavors from scientists such as Mary Dyson, Tiina Karu and many others. Collaborative science is the matrix for progress and this has become our mantra. As the journey progresses, it becomes increasingly exciting and we thank all those who share it with us.

This compilation of material reflects a distillation of sixteen years of research in the low intensity laser therapy field. The synergy created by streamlining our engineering and clinical efforts have been a significant factor in the level of success achieved. Our principal contributions reflect the manufacture of the most advanced laser therapy systems globally and the development of protocols to effectively treat a growing body of clinical pathologies.

Regulatory approvals unfortunately vary from one country to another, as do the conditions that are approved for treatment. For example, whereas one country may approve laser therapy for the treatment of lymphedema and herpes, another does not. These restrictions frequently have no basis in fact and in some instances appear to be inexplicable. Whereas we do not wish to contravene the many regulatory statutes established on a sovereign basis, we believe that any procedure that can substantially relieve a patient's pain and illness without causing harm, should be made universally available. These notes reflect the opinions of the author and members of the Meditech team.

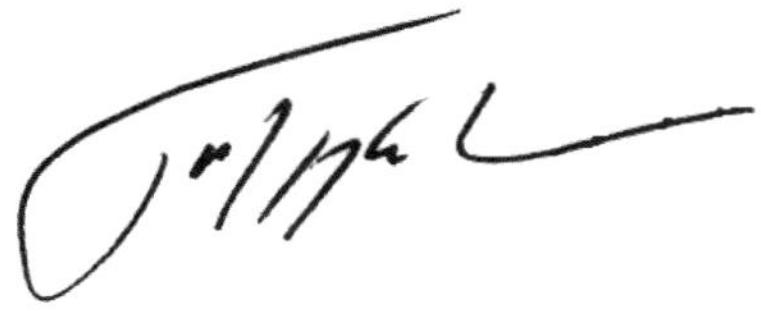

Fred Kahn, MD, FRCS(C)
Toronto, September 2005

Table of Contents

Table of Contents

Table of Contents

I Clinical Perspectives

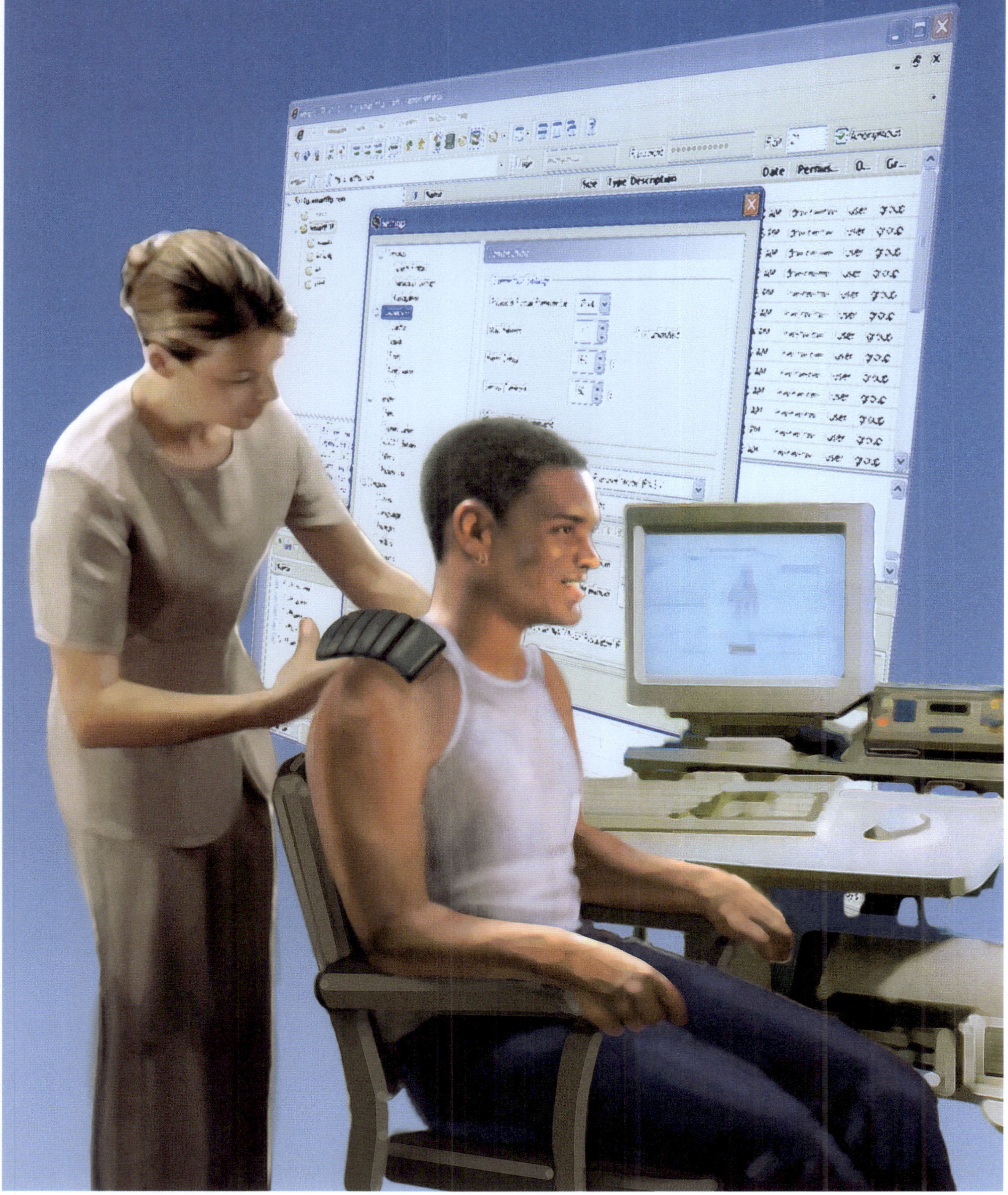

Low Intensity Laser Therapy in Clinical Practice

September 2001

Introduction

This is a definitive study based on the results of 151 consecutively discharged patients following clinical treatment with low intensity laser therapy. Low Intensity Laser Therapy was the basic platform in the therapeutic program, augmented in 50% of the cases by massage, thermal therapy and exercise. The latter were utilized to speed up the process initially, particularly in acute injuries but were not felt to be essential to the treatment program.

Historically, laser therapy has failed to gain wide acceptance in the therapeutic community for many reasons usually justifiable. Previous devices were generally poorly engineered, protocols were inappropriate and therapists were not provided with the proper education to operate the equipment. Whereas academics over the past 10 years have continued to promote additional double blind clinical trials and this is certainly commendable, in actual fact over the past decade minimal practical progress has been achieved.

At Meditech we began to recognize this problem twelve years ago at the inception of our research and in this publication share some observations, the results of our clinical approach. As we often like to quote "no patient's health status was ever improved by a test" and on occasion some have been made considerably worse. Unquestionably there is the need for continuing science and controlled studies. Ideally all tissue treated should be biopsied prior to initiating therapy and subsequently in order to accurately determine the degree of physical resolution of scar tissue, osteophytes, regeneration of cartilage and other phenomena that are discussed in the literature. Unfortunately in a normal clinical setting this is usually not possible. Notably in our studies we have evaluated patients utilizing clinical criteria that have been standard for a long period of time and are still applicable, especially if treatment and observations can be uniformly applied.

It can be stated unequivocally that in these 151 patients on completion of therapy the results are sufficiently conclusive to establish laser therapy in its proper position as the ideal therapy in treating musculo-skeletal condition, particularly when compared to symptom modulators such as ultrasound, interferential current and the use of pharmaceuticals. It should be noted that over 50% of patients in this series suffered from more than one medical problem and the majority of patients had undergone therapy varying from a matter of weeks to years to under the direction of the family physician, physiotherapist, chiropractor, neurologist, rheumatologist, orthopedic surgeon or psychologist. Analgesics, anti-inflammatory medications and cortisone had been utilized extensively in a large number of cases and many surgical procedures had been carried out, often with results that were less than desirable.

A recent review of the world literature comprising over 300 cited articles and abstracts including double blind clinical trials published between January 1998 and November 2001 reveals an overwhelming amount of evidence supporting the positive effects achieved utilizing low intensity laser therapy.

The articles that are negative have generally failed in their approach owing to inappropriate therapy. A lack of standardization, inadequate power and duration of therapy (energy density) are most frequently noted, however there exist numerous additional shortcomings. This calls to mind the work of the late Dr.

Alvan Feinstein, Sterling Professor of Medicine and Epidemiology at the Yale School of Medicine whose work I recently reviewed. Dr. Feinstein's greatest contribution was his advocacy for the information that patients can offer and the role that clinicians can play in collecting this data. In brief, Dr. Feinstein threw his weight into the issue of evidence-based-medicine versus judgmental reasoning and pathophysiological observations. He endorsed medicine-based-evidence as opposed to evidence-based-medicine. To wit the evidence will be revealed by paying close attention to the clinical status of the patient. In essence physicians must rely to greater a degree on independent clinical judgment, rather than only the observations of academic and professional journals.

At our clinic we have followed that course, customizing therapy in accordance with clinical observations based on the following criteria:

1. Reduction in pain.
2. Increase in mobility and range of motion.
3. Cessation of the use of multiple medications including analgesics, NSAIDS and cortisone.
4. The patient's general state of well being (sleep patterns, activity level, headache relief, etc.).

This requires intense effort and close term collaboration but pays immense dividends with regard to results achieved.

Results

Review Table 1. 'Compilation of Raw Data Based on the Results of 151 Consecutive Discharge Summaries'

-summarizing diagnosis, gender, age, area of treatment, number of treatments and results.

Findings

- average age of patient treated 49, average number of treatments for maximum improvement 11, overall improvement rate 89.7% (weighted average).

Table 1. Compilation of Raw Data Based on the Results of 151 Consecutive Discharge Summaries

Frequency Distribution Diagnosis	# of Cases	% of Sample	% Improvement (%) +- 0.2	Average Age	Average # of Treatments
Degenerative Osteoarthritis	45	29.8	86.1	58.4	12.3
Muscle Injuries, Tears	24	15.9	95.8	41	10.6
Rotator Cuff Injury	17	11.3	84.1	51.3	12.6
Other	17	10.6	90	41	11.2
Epicondylitis	11	7.3	99.5	52.7	8.3
Tendonitis	7	4.6	95.7	26.4	9
Trauma	5	4.0	98	54.2	5.8
Herniated Disc	5	3.3	91	45.4	17.8
Myofascial condition	4	2.6	100	46	7.5
Carpal tunnel	4	2.6	82.5	56	15.7
Plantar Fascitis	4	2.6	78.5	67.5	14
Rheumatoid Arthritis	3	2.0	90	31.6	16.3
Facet Joint Syndrome	3	2.0	100	25.3	5
Fracture	2	1.0	100	48.5	7.5
Total	**151**	**100**	**90.0**		**11.0**

Table 2. Summary of 151 Consecutively Discharged Patients

Item	#	%
Total Number of Patients	151	100
Males	94	62
Females	57	38
Average Age	49	-
Average Number of Treatments for Maximum Improvement	11.07	-
Average Percentage of Overall Improvement	-	90

Discussion

Analysis of the 151 subjects indicates that –

1. 35% of the patients fall into the category of degenerative osteoarthritis. The majority of these involved the lumbo-sacral spine and over 60% of these were accompanied by degenerative disc disease, bulging discs, nerve root compression and/ or stenosis of the spinal canal. Numerically in descending order came knees, the cervical spine, hips and ankles.

2. In excess of 35% of cases were in the sports injury sector. Individuals in this group were generally younger and the injuries healed with surprising rapidity. For example a 28-year-old NFL safety with a non-resolving tear of the biceps femoris muscle, distally involving the tendon junction had been treated for over two weeks with multiple other therapies without any improvement. This patient was restored to 100% functional capacity in asymptomatic condition after six days of consecutive treatment involving 40 minutes per session, utilizing the BioFlex system. Younger gymnasts, hockey and basketball players often with severe and long-term injuries responded in similar fashion, a feature gratifying to both patient and therapist.

3. 20% of cases were ascribed to the repetitive motion injury component. A significant percentage of these individuals work with computers and sit for long periods of time. In some instances these included rotator cuff injuries, carpal tunnel syndrome, epicondylitis and what we sometimes refer to as "the shoulder-neck-arm syndrome".

4. The remaining 10% were composed of a variety of diagnoses such as rheumatoid arthritis, acromio-clavicular joint pathology, plantar fascitis and trauma.

5. In almost every situation the biomechanical factor was active. A patient might present with severe symptoms relating to the back, hips and both knees. Through careful assessment our approach was to treat the area most severely affected. This method resolves the symptoms in most of the other areas, obviating the need for additional treatments. This can be ascribed to the compensatory biomechanical factors involved.

Conclusions

1. Low intensity laser therapy utilized as the primary therapy in the treatment of musculoskeletal problems including soft tissues and sports related injuries, arthritis and repetitive motion injuries was found to be highly effective.
2. The therapeutic process can be accelerated utilizing massage, thermal modalities, gentle stretching in the early phases and strengthening programs as the acute symptoms are alleviated.
3. Whereas we have made immense progress in both the engineering and application of this new technological approach, we expect continuing advances as our experience and knowledge increase.
4. Low intensity laser therapy appropriately customized for each individual as required can best be described as the most dramatic advance in the rehabilitation process.

Note: This study has excluded patients who for a variety of reasons failed to complete the prescribed course of treatment and those who are continuing maintenance therapy.

For References, see Bibliography

The Relevance of Laser Therapy in Current Clinical Practice

January 2003

Introduction

Over the past three decades many research groups have attempted to define the interaction between photon light and cellular structures. Few, however, have focused on the development of appropriate devices and protocols required for effective clinical therapy.

Karu, Dyson, Calderhead and many other basic researchers have clearly advanced our understanding of the above phenomena, however it was left to the clinicians and engineering disciplines to validate these theories and generate the factual evidence.

As development of the technology progressed - a work still in progress - many articles were written usually espousing a particular perspective. Three factions emerged: one, the proponents of the technology; two, those who remain perpetually undecided and lastly, the naysayers, who appear genetically opposed to any new therapy. All groups do agree on one issue however – "that further studies are required". As a result, numerous double blind clinical studies continue to be performed in addition to in vivo and in vitro laboratory experiments. Other researchers resorted to more simply devised clinical trials and observations. Unfortunately the majority of these lacked standardization of devices and reproducible protocols The field has been additionally complicated by the recent introduction of a variety of proprietary medications such as Chondroitin Sulphate, Glucosamine and a plethora of oral and topical compounds whose virtues are constantly being extolled by the manufacturing sector.

Scientific evidence of efficacy is generally shrouded in mystery, and one can never discard the all-important placebo effect. Rather than clarifying the multiple issues involved, these developments in essence serve only to further the confusion in an already cluttered field.

Annually a number of laser conferences are held at a variety of locales worldwide, signifying an ongoing interest in the technology. Numerous erudite papers are presented, but, again, these invariably end with the conclusion that, "Low Intensity Laser Therapy is a novel approach that shows promise" – with the recommendation that further studies are required to validate effectiveness. Whereas this is entirely correct from a philosophical perspective, it leads to an overwhelming level of inertia.

Requirements to be Observed

To produce conclusive studies, a number of important factors must be observed. Unfortunately, these are generally lacking, i.e.;

1. Standardized devices suitably engineered to deliver accurate reproducible irradiation dosages. These must be able to deliver frequencies, duty cycles, waveforms, pulse modulation and energy densities etc., over a wide range.
2. A significant number of patients in the various categories must be studied whether in the area of trauma, degenerative or inflammatory disease.
3. Application of the technology in consistent fashion, by therapists who are fully trained, understand anatomy, pathology and clinical medicine.
4. Notwithstanding the utilization of pre and post-therapy tissue biopsies – ideal but generally precluded by physical and ethical circumstances – results must be evaluated by definitive methods. We have found the following to be reliable.

A) Decrease in pain utilizing a visual analog scale.
B) Quantitative measurement of range of motion, mobility and function.
C) Improvement in quality of life, i.e. energy and activity levels, sleep patterns, etc.
D) Eliminating the need for pharmaceuticals and/or surgical intervention.
These criteria, carefully assessed, are acceptable indicators of the clinical status.

Medically Unexplained Symptoms

All therapists are periodically presented with patients suffering from acute/chronic pain that cannot be explained. In addition to the compilation of a thorough history and the performance of a physical examination, extensive tests including CT scans and MRI's are often performed in order to establish a diagnosis.
As Boston psychiatrist and researcher Arthur Barsky stated in a recent editorial in the Annals of Internal Medicine, "somatic and visceral symptoms have a surprisingly weak relationship to objective measures of tissue pathology". This reflects how little we know about symptom perception, processing and reporting - in other words, often we do not have a clue about what is causing the pain. Even more confusing, the definition of MUS (Medically Unexplained Symptoms) depends on who you ask.
An internist may call it functional, which means he doesn't know;
A psychiatrist may term it psychosomatic, ascribing it to the patients' state of mind,
A neurologist will term it irritation of a nerve which means it cannot be proven.
Research about MUS indicates that 20% of medical problems do not have a discernible cause. Moreover, people with MUS on average spend 3.5 days per month in bed.

In our practice, most pain can be explained applying the standard medical approach. We listen to the patient, perform an extensive physical examination and utilize test procedures as indicated. Over 70% of our patient population is referred and have already been studied with varying degrees of enthusiasm by a number of healthcare professionals. The majority have utilized an extensive array of medications from 1 to 12 in number and not infrequently in excess of 30 analgesics on a daily basis. Others have been subjected to a variety of surgical procedures, often with less than desirable results.

Table 3. Distribution of Conditions among 286 Consecutively Discharged Patients

Conditions	Number of Cases	Percentage of Cases	Average Number of Treatments	Percentage Overall Improvement
Degenerative Conditions	108	38.3	11.5	87.6
Sports Injuries	89	31.4	7.8	96
Trauma	48	14.8	8.9	93
Repetitive Motion Injuries	35	12.3	10.7	88.7
Other	6	3.2	11.1	91.1
Total	**286**	**100**	**9.7**	**91.1**

Table 4. Age Distribution (n=286 patients)

Item	Value	
Age Distribution	Youngest = 7 years	Oldest = 91 years
Mean Age	52.5 years	

Table 5. Improvement Rate (n=286 patients)

Item	Value
Significant Improvement: Cure Rate	91 %
Overall Average Number of Treatments	9.7

Table 6. Improvement Range (n=286 patients)

Range	Number of Cases	Percentage of Total
0 - 5%	0	0
6 - 25%	4	1.4
26 - 50%	6	2.1
51 - 75%	37	12.9
76 - 100%	37	83.6
	239	100

Table 7. Gender Distribution (n=286 patients)

Gender	Number of Cases	Percentage of Cases
Males	170	59.4
Females	116	40.6

Discussion

In this, the second in a series of three proposed papers in support of the intelligent application of Low Intensity Laser Therapy, 286 consecutive discharged patients are presented. The significant improvement / cure rate is somewhat higher, compared to the 151 reported in our first publication in this series, produced in September 2001. Moreover, the average number of treatments has been reduced by 12%. This can be attributed to protocol selection and application.

As the patient load in our clinic increases, we note a commensurate increase in the number of back problems, degenerative arthritis and sports injuries. Surveys indicate that this is based on patient and physician referrals, the result of superior treatment outcomes. Moreover athletes both at the high performance amateur and professional level are highly motivated to return to activity and rapidly develop dependence on this dramatic therapeutic approach.

Conclusion

Once again, one can only state that Low Intensity Laser Therapy judiciously applied produces results unequaled by other technologies if the appropriate criteria are observed. Furthermore, it reinforces the fact that Low Intensity Laser Therapy is the therapy of choice in the treatment of musculoskeletal pathologies.

For References, see Bibliography.

The Role of Low Intensity Laser in the Maintenance of Optimal Health

A review of 576 Consecutive Patient Discharges at the Meditech Clinic.
November 2003

Introduction

The best preventative medicine predicating long life is to be born with good genes. Unfortunately this remains beyond our personal control. At the same time a healthy lifestyle is no less important. This incorporates a number of factors that are under our control and some guidelines are provided.

1. Probably the most important and least recognized is the avoidance of stress and for further enlightenment I refer the reader to the work of Hans Selye who first recognized the impact of this factor. In the era of the technological revolution, dramatic changes in lifestyle and the workplace, the negative influence of stress is increasing exponentially at an alarming rate. When counseling patients who recognize the adverse influence of this widely prevalent condition I recommend that they change careers, retire or move to rural communities where lifestyle pressures are diminished.

2. The ingestion of a balanced diet cannot be overlooked. Nutritionists often count calories which from a practical point of view is a course that may be difficult to follow. A diet based on natural components such as fresh vegetables, fruit, cereals and fish is best from a broad perspective. All processed and refined foods and those with additives and preservatives should be studiously avoided.

3. Vitamin and mineral supplements are required regardless of the dietary intake. These include vitamins B, C and E along with small amounts of zinc, selenium, magnesium and a number of other components. Again, these should be ingested in proper amounts on a daily basis no matter how balanced the diet and once again the rule of moderation is the best guide.

4. A regular exercise program geared to the individual's needs and capabilities is also essential. The platform should consist of a daily minimum workout of thirty minutes. Swimming is unquestionably the best all around exercise both from the cardiovascular and muscle toning perspective. Moreover it avoids trauma to the musculoskeletal system. I invariably cringe when I see runners on paved roads, breathing air that almost visually reveals the multiple environmental contaminants present.

   The increasing use of weights and exercise machines creates many problems that can easily be avoided particularly in the aging population. Personal trainers can be helpful but often set goals and standards for their clients that are inappropriate. Excessive/obsessive exercise programs erase the benefit that can be attained by a more moderate approach. Whereas more intensive programs need to be incorporated in the regime of professional and high level amateur athletes, with individuals over 50 who essentially wish to maintain their physical status, the approach should be denoted by moderation. Walking, swimming, isometric and stretching exercises, yoga, pilates and low impact activities are preferred methods.

5. Tobacco products must be avoided and alcohol ingestion should be limited.

   Most individuals are sufficiently intelligent to recognize that nature cures many illnesses, however, in some situations a rigid medical regime is required i.e. cancer, diabetes, hypertension, etc. Taking this one step further it becomes readily apparent that therapeutic approaches that stimulate natural processes are clearly the most appropriate in dealing with many healthcare problems where no specific therapy exists.

Surgery is a court of last resort, although there are many conditions where this approach is preferable. On the other hand surgical procedures are sometimes contraindicated, particularly if performed for the relief of pain without alternative therapies having been adequately considered or implemented. This is by no means an indictment of surgical intervention. Still, regardless of the surgeon's capabilities or the quality of the individual's tissues, results achieved with this approach are often less than optimal. Time and nature assisted by intelligent non-invasive therapies often produce a more ideal result.

Probably the most deleterious aspect of modern medicine is the almost relentless utilization by healthcare practitioners of a wide variety of pharmaceuticals, essentially to treat symptoms. Again, most physicians are well intentioned but in an atmosphere filled with stress, the interference and practice methodology imposed by governments, insurance companies, healthcare plans, audits, codes and other regulatory bodies, often too little time is available for quality patient care, i.e. the time to take a complete history, perform a thorough physical examination and order appropriate tests with a subsequent review in order to establish the correct diagnosis and the development of the proper therapeutic approach.

In current practice there appears to be a rush both by the patient and the physician for the "quick fix" i.e. instant gratification. This often-reflex type activity results in masking serious problems and over-medication particularly of the elderly, a most pernicious aspect of medical practice today. When symptoms are treated with pharmaceuticals, frequently other symptoms result and additional medications are utilized resulting in a total imbalance of the homeostatic biological state. Moreover, drugs are frequently addictive and have a significant negative effect on the natural immune system of the individual. This is an alarming problem particularly among seniors, psychiatric patients and those patients suffering from chronic conditions, including the arthritides. Unquestionably this is one of the most serious problems confronting physicians today; unfortunately this practice has become the standard accepted approach. Psychomimetic, antilipid and NSAID drugs are utilized almost indiscriminately and often shorten the life of the patient rather than relieving the ongoing disease process, aside from causing gastrointestinal hemorrhage, aplastic anemic, liver disease, and possible malignancies along with other disastrous side effects. Under these circumstances, it is appropriate if not urgent for leaders in medicine to more enthusiastically embrace the use of the simple preventative measures outlined and include therapies such as Low Intensity Laser Therapy, which delivers many benefits without any negative side effects. Aside from the many entities that can be safely and effectively treated one cannot overlook the positive effect on the body's immune response. At this time, the technology has clearly established its dramatic effectiveness in the treatment of many disease processes and can be widely applied in a safe manner.
This article presents the results of 576 consecutive patient discharges at the Meditech Clinic and is the third article in a trilogy designed to attest to the safe and effective use of this therapy. It brings to a total of 1,013 consecutive patient discharges studied, once again proving its dramatic impact. See Tables 8 – 12.

Table 8. Distribution of Pathologies (n=576 patients)

Conditions	Number of Cases	Percentage of Cases	Average Number of Treatments	Percentage Overall Improvement
Degenerative Conditions	140	24.3	11.2	88.34
Repetitive Stress	93	16.1	9.6	94.30
Trauma	66	11.4	9.4	94.50
Sports Injuries	258	44.7	9.1	96.[illegible]1
Other	19	3.2	7.5	96.31
Total	**576**	**100**	**9.68**	**93.72**

Table 9. Overview of Cases Studied (n=576 patients)

Item	Data
Total Number of Cases	576 Patients
Average Number of Treatments per Patient	9.68 Treatments
Percentage Overall Improvement	93.6% Improvement*

*Based on ROM/VAS/Reduction in Medication/Patient Declaration

Table 10. Gender Distribution (n=576 patients)

Gender	Number of Cases	Percentage of Cases
Males	316	54.9
Females	260	45.1

Table 11. Age Distribution (n=576 patients)

Age	Number of Cases	Percentage of Cases
0 to 15	10	1.5
16 to 30	37	6.2
31 to 45	118	20.3
46 to 60	214	37.1
61 to 75	166	28.6
76 to 88	31	5.2

Table 12. Pathologies, Age and Gender Spread (n=576 patients)

Conditions	Number of Cases	Average Age	Male Percentage (#)	Female Percentage (#)	Percentage of Improvement
Degenerative	140	65.3	40% (56)	60% (84)	88.3
Repetitive Stress	93	51.6	42% (39)	58% (54)	94.3
Trauma	66	49.9	41% (27)	59% (39)	96.0
Sports Injuries	258	47.6	71% (183)	29% (75)	91.1
Other	19	54.2	63% (12)	37% (7)	96.3
Total	**576**				**93.72**

Conclusion

As the accompanying data will demonstrate, the majority of cases involve sports injuries, trauma, arthritis and repetitive motion injuries. The significant improvement/cure rate is in excess of 90% after an average 9.68 treatments. Once again the case for the use of Low Intensity Laser Therapy has been clearly established and the following conclusions derived.

1. Modern medicine can benefit significantly with the wider adaptation of Low Intensity Laser Therapy in the treatment many pathological conditions.

2. It would be appropriate for all practitioners of medicine to review current methods of practice and institute changes minimizing the utilization of pharmaceuticals and the application of superior alternative methods.

3. A complete re-evaluation of the use of pharmaceuticals with regard to benefits versus dangers should be applied. In our experience almost without exception patients are on 2-12 medications often in copious amounts and the negative aspect of this practice is readily apparent.

4. Lifestyle and preventative medicine should be key essentials consistent with good medical practice along with the incorporation of improved and safer technologies.

5. This approach could beneficially revolutionize current healthcare both from an economic and result-oriented basis.

For References, see Bibliography.

Table 13. Summary of the clinical analysis of 1013 consecutively discharged patients (3 Studies).

Study	***#1***	***#2***	***#3***
# of Cases Evaluated	***151***	***286***	***576***
Avg # Tx's	11.1	9.7	9.68
% Improvement	90	91.1	93.6
Case Breakdown	***# of Cases***		
Sports Injury	22	89	258
Degenerative	48	108	140
Repetitive Stress	28	35	93
Trauma	36	48	66
Other	17	6	19
Total	***151***	***286***	***576***
% Improvement			
Degenerative	86.3	87.6	88.3
Repetitive Stress	87.8	88.7	94.3
Trauma	95.6	93	96
Sports Injury	94.4	96	96.1
Other	90	91.1	96.3
SUM	***90***	***91.1***	***93.6***
Average # Tx's			
Degenerative	12.55	11.5	11.31
Repetitive Stress	11.5	10.7	9.59
Trauma	10.7	8.9	9.37
Sports Injury	9.34	7.8	9.17
Other	11.2	11.1	7.5
SUM	***11***	***9.7***	***9.68***

Low Intensity Laser Therapy in the Treatment of Juvenile Rheumatoid Arthritis

Clinical Abstract, January 2000

History

Case Study is that of a 17-year-old female high school student who has had progressive rheumatoid arthritis diagnosed at age 13. The disease is generalized, but the most severe symptoms relate to the hands and most particularly the digits. The diagnosis was established by her pediatrician and she has been under the care of rheumatologists since age 14. A number of pharmaceutical regimes have been utilized including Tetracycline, Naprosyn, Plaquenil, and Voltaren, often in combination. The suggestion was made to add Methotrexate to the regimen in October 1999. The patient and her family resisted this approach and came to our clinic asking for evaluation and assistance in therapy

Physical Examination

At the time of presentation in October 1999, the patient revealed significant edema of the digits particularly from digits 2 to 5 inclusive. The fingers had a "sausage like" appearance bilaterally. The metacarpal phalangeal joints and the interphalangeal joints were most severely affected. Strength bilaterally was substantially diminished from the expected norm and measured 12 Kg. on the right and 10.5 on the left using the Asimow dynamometer. She could barely touch her fingertips to her palm due to edema and pain.

Treatment

Low Intensity Laser Therapy was initiated on a three times per week basis and was adhered to with the exception of several week-long holidays and school examinations. The regimen utilized, incorporated a combination of BioFlex treatment arrays including the R-750, the IR-1500 and the IR-75 laser probe. This was consistently applied over a three month period. When noticeable improvement occurred, treatments were reduced to twice per week. Therapy was eventually cut back to once per week and the patient was discharged at the end of June. She will be observed periodically to determine whether she maintains her dramatic improvement. It should be noted that a total of 28 treatments were applied.

Current Status

(6 month's post cessation of treatments)
The patient's hands and fingers are relatively normal in appearance with only minimal thickening at the proximal interphalangeal joints. Strength on the right has improved to 16 Kg. on the right and 14 Kg. on the left (the patient is right handed). She is able to make a fist without restriction of mobility and no pain exists. In January of this year, the patient's medications were reduced on a weekly basis and since April she has not taken any medications whatsoever. At this time, the patient is asymptomatic, has full range of motion, has no discernable cosmetic deficit and requires no therapy.

Table 14. Treatment Regime Followed (Rheumatoid Arthritis)
Areas: MP and IP, digits 2 to 5 inclusive.

Head	Frequency	Duty Cycle	Time/Area	Energy Density
LS-R 750	CW		5 min/hand	3.00 J/cm^2
LS-I 1500	1000 Hz	70 %	6 min/hand	5.04 J/cm^2
LD-I 75	CW		15 sec for 3 points/joint	33.75 J/cm^2

Figure 1. a) and b)

a) Palmar View of Hand. Dorsal aspect presents better access to the joints for laser therapy. However palmar approach may also be useful.

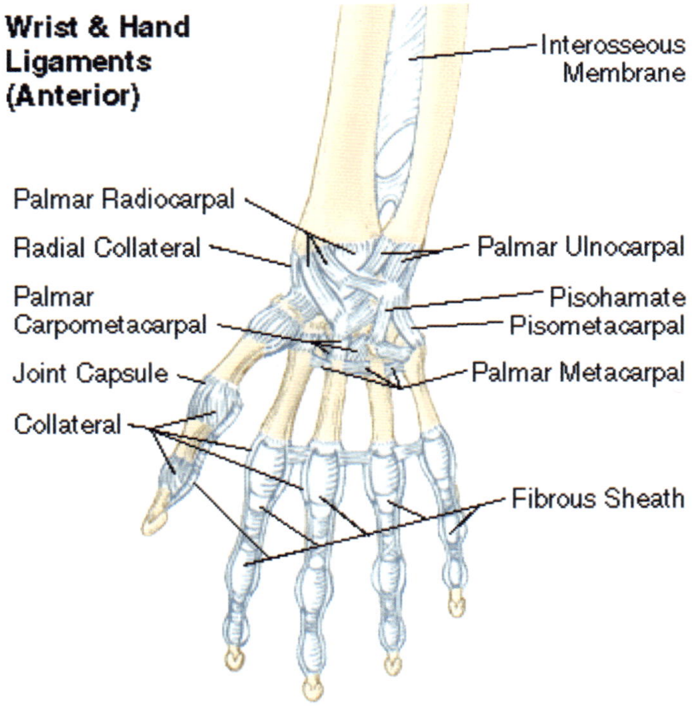

b) The Treatment Arrays (LS- R 750 & LS- I 1500) cover the entire hand and the Laser Probe (LD I 75) is directed specifically to the individual joints presenting the most severe pathology. Two stages (I &II) of treatment were applied dorsally and one stage (III) over the palmar aspect

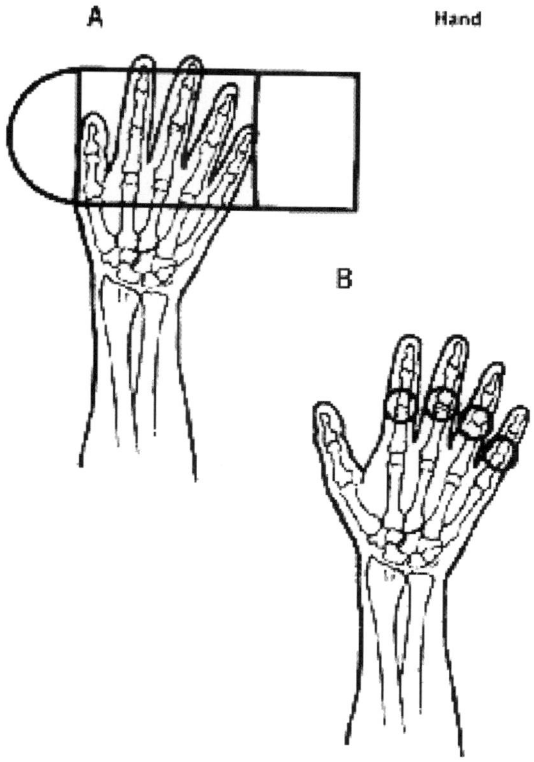

Conclusion

Low Intensity Laser Therapy is highly effective in the treatment of Rheumatoid Arthritis. This has been substantiated by a study at the Department of Rehabilitative Sciences at the University of Ulster.

For References, see Bibliography.

Low Intensity Laser Therapy in the Treatment of Periphero-Arterial Occlusive Disease

June 2004

This study consists of three patients, two of whom had previously been subjected to amputation of a lower extremity and were facing a similar situation at time of presentation in March 2004. The first two cases had suffered from a longstanding history of arterial insufficiency, accompanied by multiple dermal ulcers.

In each instance, the forefoot was deeply cyanotic and edematous, the mid foot demonstrated violent erythema and the feet were cold to the touch. There was a history of unrelenting pain and inability to sleep. Symptoms were being managed by the utilization of multiple pharmaceuticals including analgesics, medications for sleep and depression, along with aggressive oral and intravenous antibiotic therapy, and various ointments applied locally.

Discussion of Progress

In all cases, following two treatments of Low Intensity Laser Therapy over consecutive days, the feet became relatively warm and pain diminished markedly along with the cyanosis and erythema. The mobility of the feet and toes was largely restored and the extremities were no longer deemed to be in jeopardy.

Method of Treatment

Laser was applied over the lower spinal cord including the nerve roots, in addition to the autonomic nervous system and the ganglia. It should be noted that the autonomic nervous system has significant systemic effects on tissue, specifically, an increase in:

Arterial pressure.

Blood flow to active muscles.

Rate of basal cellular metabolism throughout the body.

Blood glucose concentration.

Gycolysis in the liver and muscle.

Preganglionic motor neurons of sympathetic nerve fibers originate in the spinal cord between cord segments T1 and L2, passing via the sympathetic ganglia chain to synapse with the postganglionic neurons in the tissue and organs of the body. This explains the decision to treat the sympathetic and central nervous system which regulate the vascular structures of the lower extremities.

Low Intensity Laser Therapy was also applied to the tissues locally. It has been well documented that laser has significant anti-inflammatory and analgesic effects in addition to stimulating angiogenesis.

Treatments were applied initially for 3 consecutive days and subsequently on alternate days until a state of stability had occurred and the limbs were felt to be satisfactorily healed to sustain weightbearing. Medications were gradually discontinued with the exception of insulin injections in the diabetic situation. The ulcer on the heel of the diabetic patient had decreased in size by 70% and was healing satisfactorily after 2 weeks of treatment. All other ulcers had healed almost completely.

Figure 2. Case Profile 1: Buergers Disease (Thromboangiitis Obliterans)

A retired property manager who had been confined to a wheelchair for over one year. Prior to presenting at the Meditech Clinic his left leg had been amputated and he was unemployed for one year. Following treatment the foot was warm to touch and ready for weight bearing.

Diagnosis:

Buergers Disease (Thromboangiitis Obliterans)

Duration of Symptoms:

Several years including long term conventional therapy i.e. analgesics, vasodilators, antidepressants, sleeping medications; localized wound care consisting of anti-inflammatories and antibiotic ointments.

Amputation of left leg in April 2003.

Treatment:

Laser, saline compresses, ulcers cleansed with hydrogen peroxide

Initial

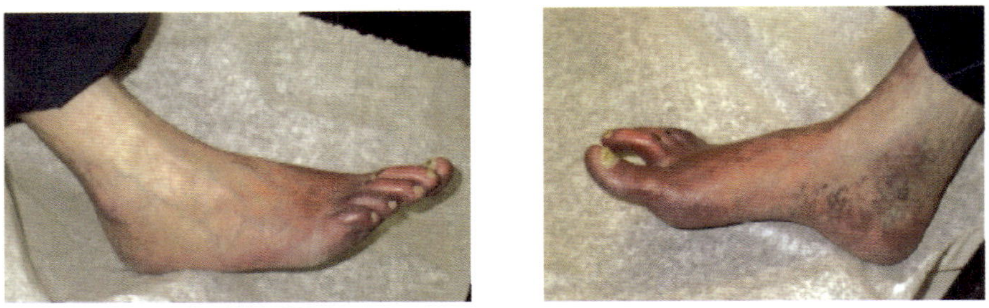

Intermediate

2 days after initiating treatment

- foot no longer in jeopardy
- improved arterial circulation and venous filling

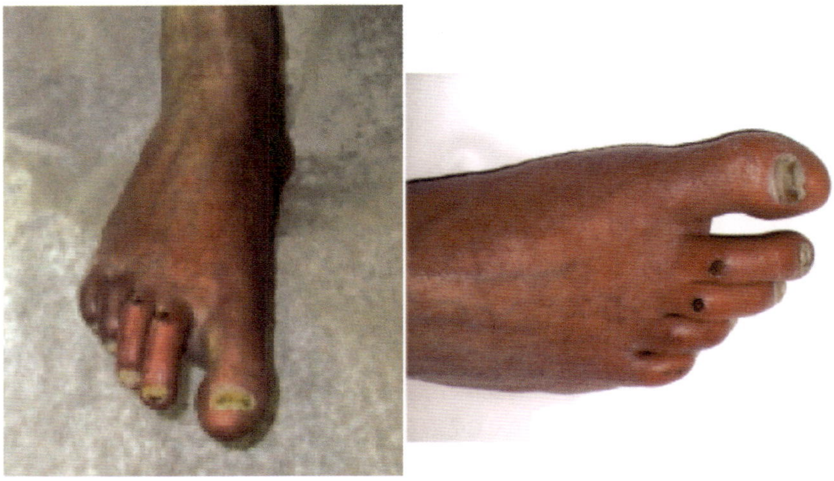

Final

12 treatments over 3 weeks

- colour normal
- one ulcer totally healed
- 2nd ulcer almost healed
- foot warm to touch
- ready for weight bearing

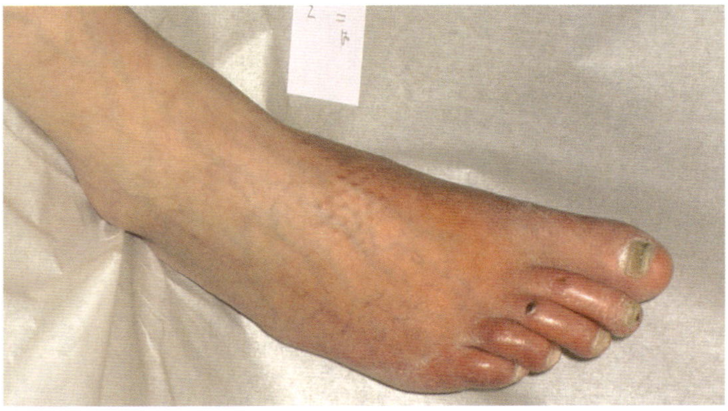

Figure 3. Case Profile 2: Diabetes Mellitus with Advanced Atherosclerosis

A semi-retired manager of a delivery business who had minimum mobility due to intermittent claudication and pain in his foot. Prior to presenting at the Meditech Clinic his right leg had been amputated and he was suffering through severe depression as well as anger and fear that his left leg would be amputated. Following treatment, six of eight ulcers had healed and he was weight bearing comfortably.

Diagnosis:

Diabetes Mellitus with advanced atherosclerosis

Duration of Symptoms:

Several years including long term conventional therapy i.e. antibiotics (Ceftzidime IV and Clindamycin orally), Altace, insulin injections twice daily, debridement by home care daily, dressings and utilization of copious amounts of antibiotic/anti-inflammatory ointments.
Amputation of right leg in May 1999
Amputation of left 5th toe in September 1999
Bilateral femero-popliteal bypass grafts in 1998
Penile implant 1984

Treatment:

Laser, saline compresses, ulcers cleansed with hydrogen peroxide

Initial

- Photos (1-4) demonstrating dermal ulcers of diabetic extremity.

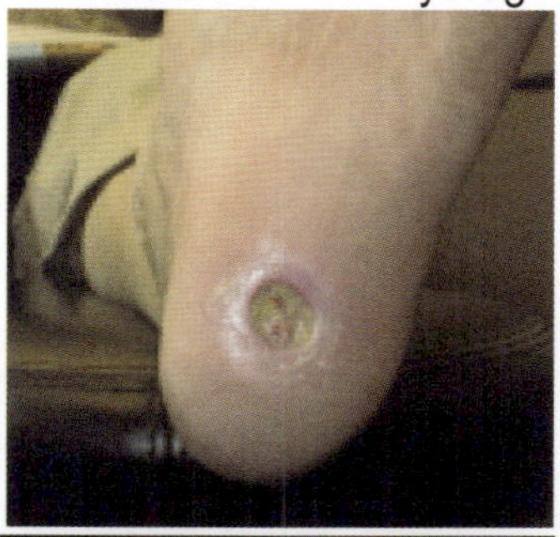

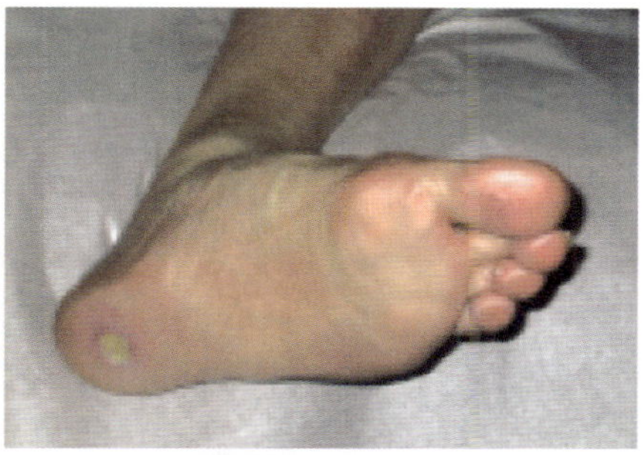

Interim

- Five days after initiating treatment, ulcers (4) on forefoot healing rapidly.

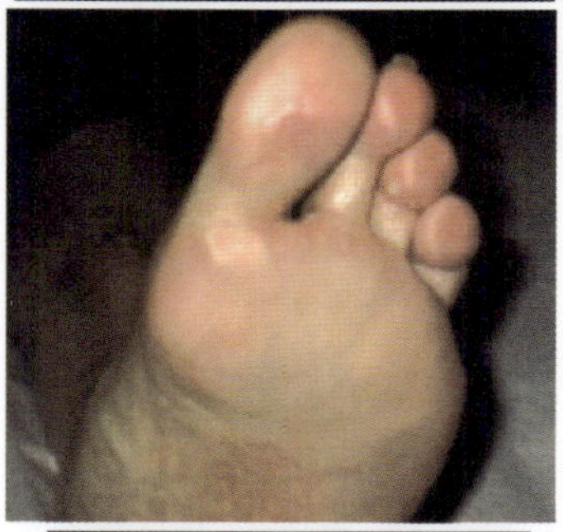

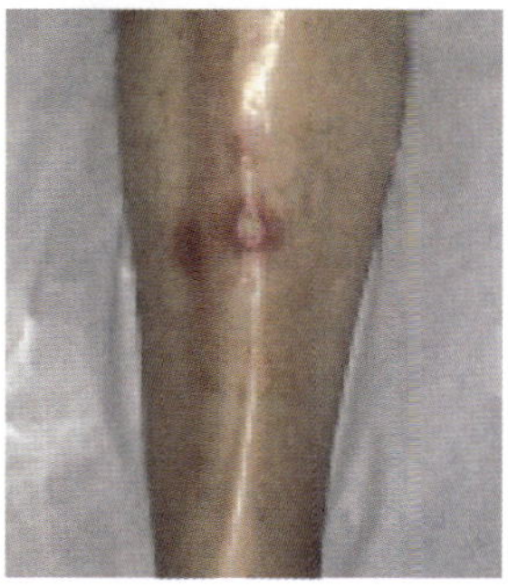

10 treatments over two weeks

- colour normal
- improved circulation
- all ulcers (initially 8) except 1 on anterior tibia and heel, resolved
- weight bearing comfortably

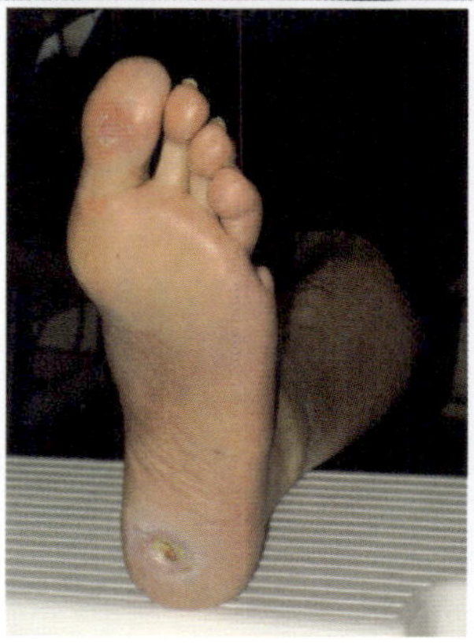

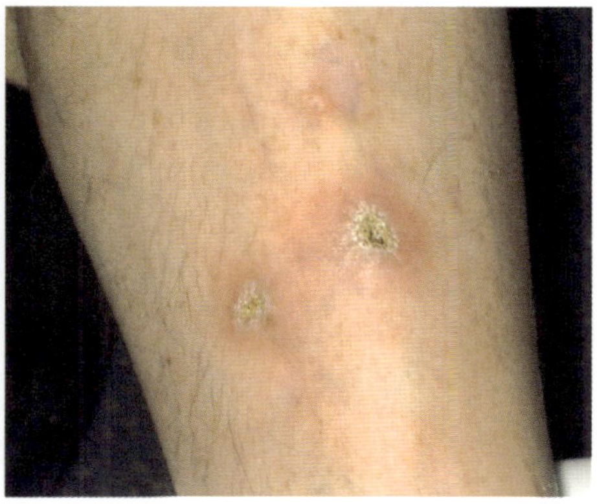

Figure 4. Case Profile 3. Periphero-Arterial Occlusive Disease (frostbite):
The patient was an 86 year old podiatrist who had periphero-arterial occlusive disease that created a pre-gangrenous status in his foot. The problem had been complicated by severe frostbite of his toes during a prior skiing excursion. He was advised that partial amputation would be necessary. The patient decided to find alternative therapy and presented at our clinic. Following treatment the foot had returned to normal colour and temperature and was asymptomatic.

Diagnosis:

Periphero-Arterial Occlusive Disease

Duration of Symptoms:

6 months prior to presenting at the Meditech Clinic

Treatment:

5 daily treatments over one week

Initial

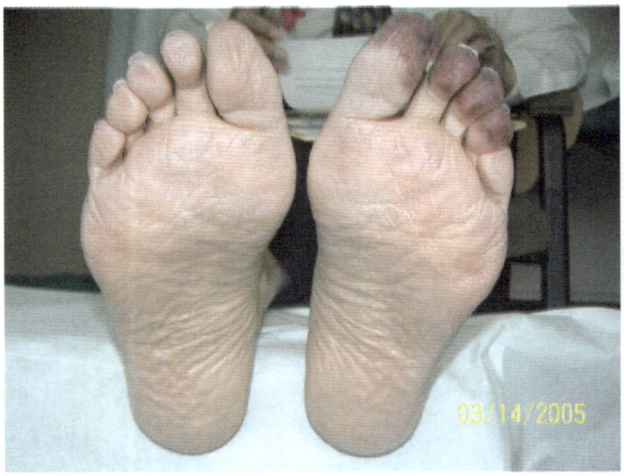

Final

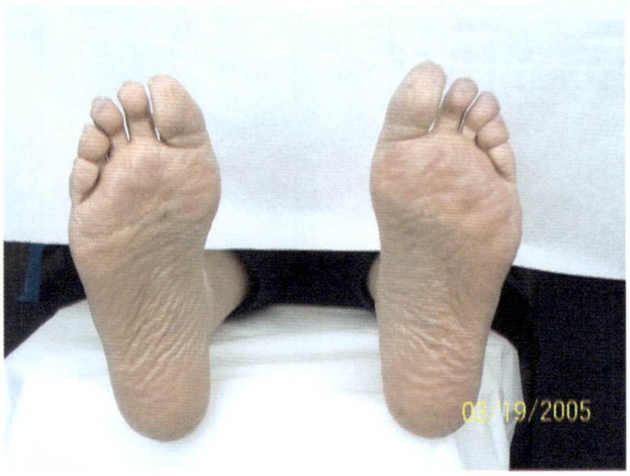

After 5 consecutive days of laser therapy

Status maintained 1 year post conclusion of treatment

Figure 5. Case Profile 4: Periphero-Arterial Occlusive Disease (Crushing injury)
Following intensive laser therapy to the lumbosacral spine and the left lower extremity, particularly the knee, left gastroc and forefoot, all problems resolved to the degree where there is no clinical evidence of vascular impairment and the patient is ambulating without the use of crutches. He has also ceased to take any analgesics after 35 years of continued use.

Diagnosis:

1. Degenerative osteoarthritis lumbosacral spine, left knee and ankle.
2. Periphero-arterial occlusive disease left lower extremity

Physical Findings:

Forefoot cold, cyanotic and immobile
Severe tenderness over left lateral gastrocnemius

Duration of Symptoms:

Crushing injury of left lower extremity; leg caught between two automobiles 35 years ago. Since that time the patient has chronic/acute pain and is only able to ambulate to a limited degree. He has utilized in excess of 25 analgesics daily including Percocet, OxyContin, Toradol, etc He initially presented with severe pain in the left calf and foot; also, significant chronic pain in the lumbosacral spine. Only able to walk short distances with crutches, prior to treatment.

Treatments:

12 treatments over 3 weeks

Initial

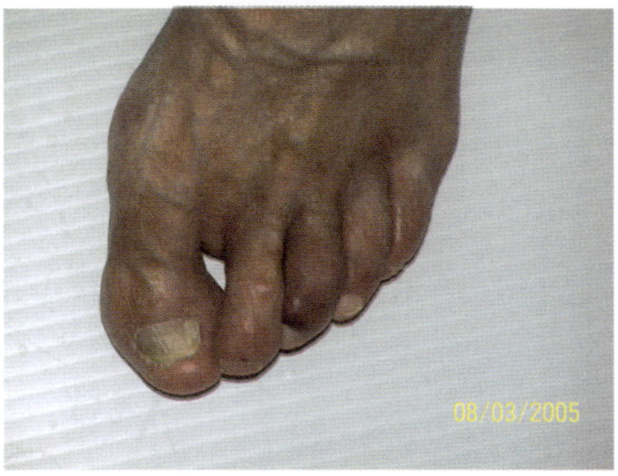

Intermediate

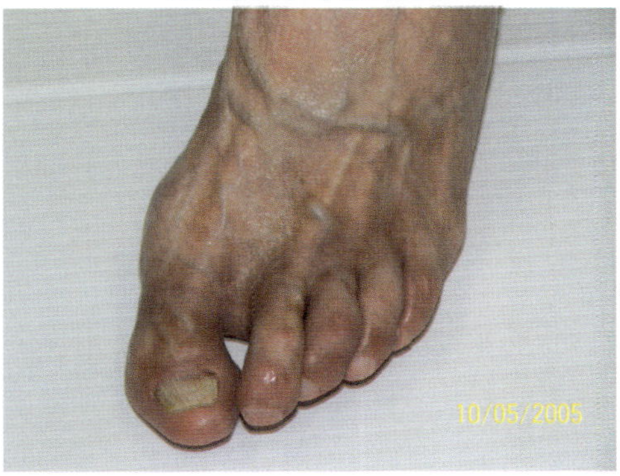

Final

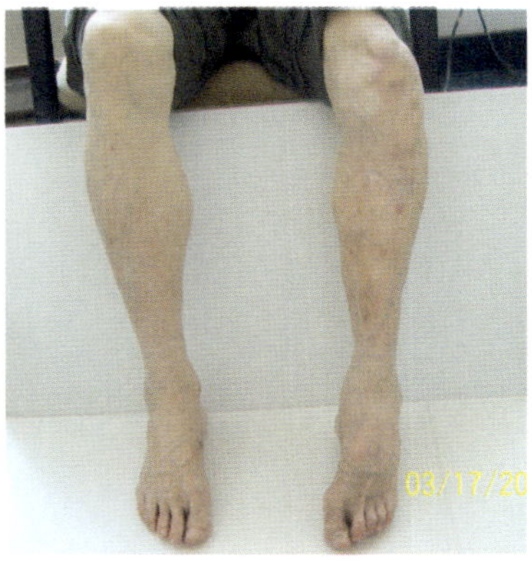

This slide demonstrates the extensive trauma to the left lower extremity 35 years earlier.

Conclusions

These cases illustrate the dramatic effectiveness of Low Intensity Laser Thearpy in the treatment of Periphero-Arterial Occlusive Disease.

Moreover, they indicate the need for practitioners to re-evaluate the current therapeutic approach based on the use of high doses of antibiotics, analgesics, vasodilators, anti-inflammatory agents and local ointments applied to the ulcers. It is clear that this approach is totally ineffective and indeed, may be counterproductive as ulcers continued to enlarge despite aggressive drug therapy.

It appears based on the evidence that the previous amputations may have been avoidable.

A superior approach of the treatment of arterio-vascular occlusive disease is demonstrated and the recommendation is that it should be more widely employed.

For References, see Bibliography

Lymphedema: A Review and Case Profiles

October 2004

Lymphedema of the extremities remains a therapeutic challenge. As a result many different treatments have been devised but none have been routinely effective.

Two types of lymphedema occur, primary and secondary. Primary lymphedema is rare, the result of a congenital abnormality of the lymphatic system. Secondary lymphedema, the most common form, may be acute or chronic. It results from obstruction or interruption of the lymphatic channels. Fluids and proteins, transudate from cells or exudate from both lymphatic and vascular channels collects in the superficial connective tissues and fails to be absorbed by the lymphatic system. Duration varies from weeks to years.

The acute form generally follows trauma and is easily resolved by conventional methods. The chronic version is a more vexing problem, only minimally improved by existing technologies with rapid recurrence when therapy ceases. Chronic lymphedema most frequently occurs post-mastectomy or subsequent to a variety of other surgical procedures that involve resection of the lymph channels and nodes. It can also be a complication secondary to congestive heart failure, chronic liver disease, thrombophlebitis, systemic infections and gravitational dependency. In its late stages it is characterized by firm induration with accompanying cyanosis as arterial compression occurs.

Table #15. Lymphedema Etiology

Acute	Chronic
• Trauma	• Thrombophlebitis
• Surgery	• Congestive Cardiac Failure
• Burns	• Immobilization
	• Dependency
	• Post Radiation
	• Renal Failure
	• Hepatic Disease
	• Systemic Infection
	• Developmental

Conventional Therapies

1. Elevation of extremity above level of heart	
2. Variety of compression techniques	Pumps
	Bandages
	Fitted garments
3. Manual Procedures	Massage
	Compression

It should be noted that there is no effective drug therapy available. Diuretics are frequently utilized but not recommended for long term use. The above listed conventional therapies do not provide long term solutions. Outcomes are usually limited at best and require prolonged periods of treatment without permanent relief or cure.

Case Profile #1

80 year old male.

Duration
3 to 4 years. Progressive in nature.

Etiology
Post harvesting long saphenous vein (coronary bypass procedure)
Gravitational dependency
Recurrent congestive heart failure

Findings
Initially affected extremity circumference mid-calf 6 cm greater than opposite side
Firm non-pitting induration
Moderate cyanosis
Poor venous filling
No palpable arterial pulse distal to femoral pulse

Treatment
Ten one-hour sessions over a four week period utilizing the BioFlex Low Intensity Laser Therapy System.
Treatment was applied over the sympathetic nervous system and locally.

Outcome

Objective
Mid-calf circumference same as opposite side
Resolution of cyanosis and induration
Restoration of venous filling and peripheral arterial pulses
Normal skin temperature

Subjective
Absence of sensation of heaviness, chronic aching
Activity level restored to normal
No regression or recurrence four months post-cessation of treatment.

Figure 6. Case Profile #1. Lymphedema Prior to and Following Treatment with LILT.

Initial | **Final**

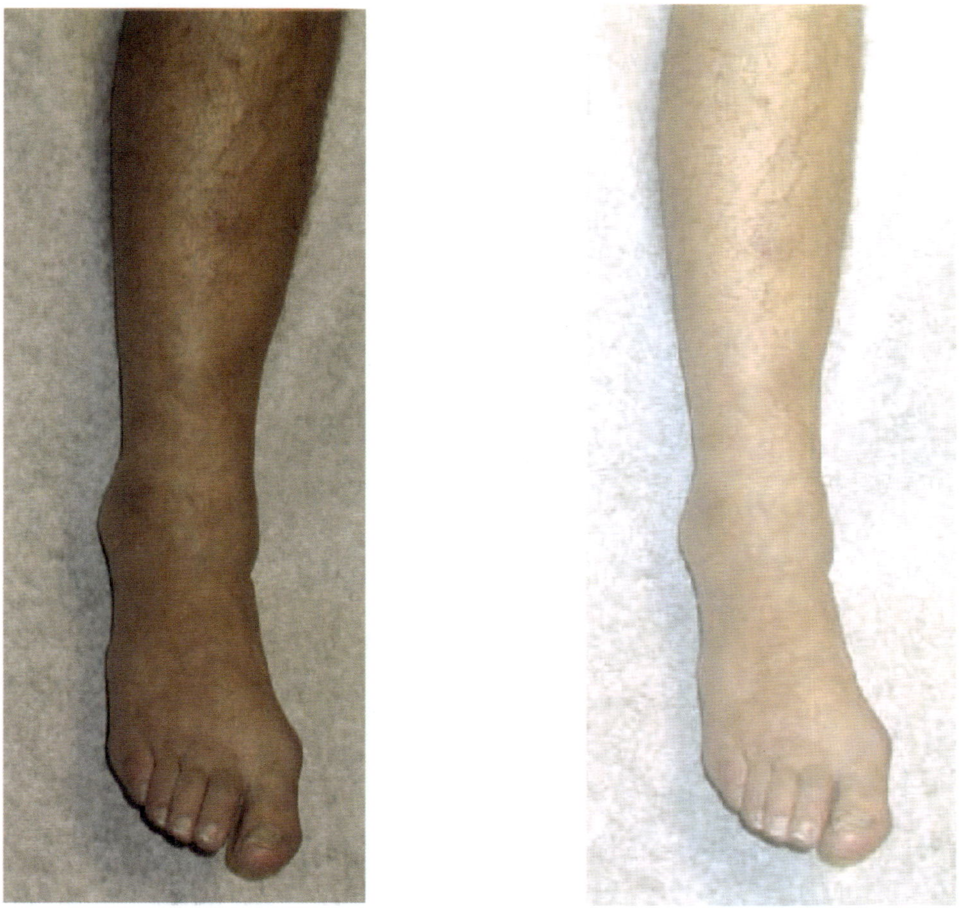

After 10 Treatments

- Cyanosis and induration gone
- Good venous filling
- Mid-calf diameter same as left

Case Profile #2

58 year old female

Duration

Liver transplant in1986 precipitated by hepatitis and hepatic failure

Diagnosis

Chronic lymphedema of left lower extremity with accompanying cellulitis

Etiology

Thrombophlebitis of deep veins
Anti-rejection medications
Hypoalbuminemia
Gravitational dependency

Findings

Initially right leg mid-calf circumference – 35 cm
Left leg mid-calf circumference – 43 cm

Treatment

Nine one-hour sessions over three weeks using BioFlex Low Intensity Laser Therapy System in circumferential manner.

Outcome

Left leg mid-calf circumference – 38 cm
Cellulitis 90% resolved without antibiotics
(Note - At this time patient moved away and is continuing treatment at another facility using the BioFlex System.)

Figure 7. Case Profile # 2. Lymphedema Prior to and Following Treatment with LILT.

Initial

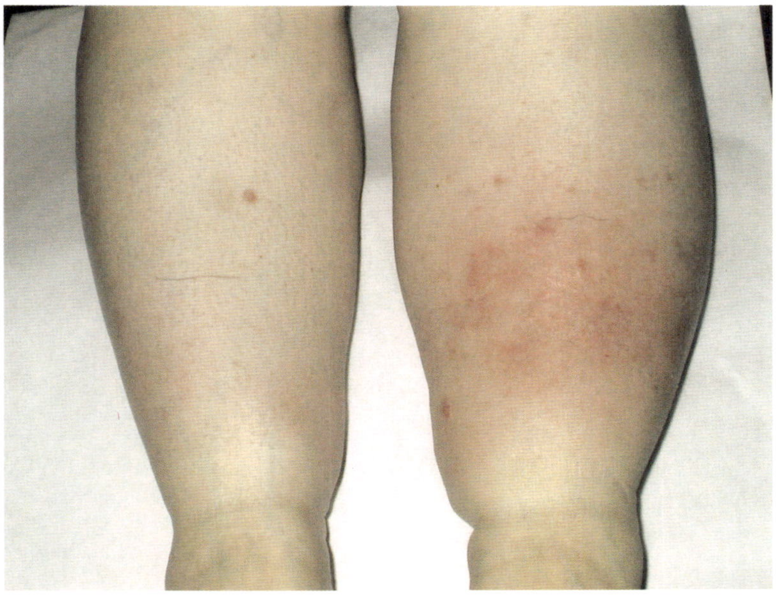

Intermediate

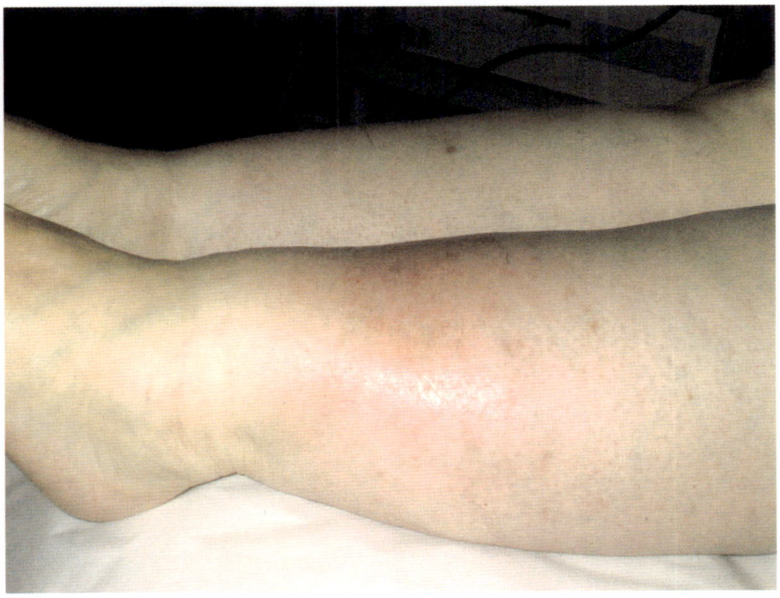

After 9 treatments
(mid calf diameter reduced 6 cm)
(Patient relocated and continued treatment at another clinic)

Discussion

Large surface treatment arrays are applied in circumferential fashion to the affected areas. Often in these situations arterial circulation is compromised; in order to relieve this and enhance reduction of the edema, Low Intensity Laser Therapy may also be applied to the appropriate dermatomes of the spinal column, resulting in a sympathectomy-type effect. We utilize this technique in the treatment of edema in both the upper and lower extremities. This accelerates resolution of the pathology and its ensuing complications.

Conclusion

Low intensity laser therapy is effective in the treatment of both acute and chronic lymphedema. Notwithstanding duration of the condition in our experience response is rapid with total elimination of the problem in less than four weeks.

The Bio-Flex Low Intensity Laser Therapy System is therefore recommended as the therapy of choice in treating lymphedema.

For References, see Bibliography.

Wound Healing

March 2005

The management of wounds has been a challenge to a variety of medical disciplines since time immemorial.

Dermatologists, physiatrists, physiotherapists and naturopaths at various times have focused their therapeutic efforts on solving these complex medical conditions without achieving a significant degree of success. Indeed, prior to this time no simple or permanent solution has been found.

To address this issue one must consider causation, environmental factors and the therapeutic methodologies currently employed.

Aside from the economic impact, morbidity and mortality implications, the need for effective therapeutic solutions is paramount at this point in time.

Etiological Factors:

1. Systemic diseases - diabetes, Buerger's disease, etc.
2. Pressure ulcers – (bedsores)
3. Arteriosclerosis - periphero-vascular occlusive disease (lack of oxygenation)
4. Thrombophlebitis - inadequate venous drainage
5. Chronic lymphedema – compression of arteries.
6. Injuries - lacerations, contusions
7. Thermal burns
8. Surgical wounds
9. Infections - bacterial (anaerobic environment; osteomyelitis)

If wound healing is to occur, all negative factors in the environment must be eradicated or controlled. Although wounds may start at deeper levels, healing occurs from the periphery and growth is centrally directed (epithelization). Once closure is achieved infection disappears and modeling will continue. If the negative factors are controlled 25% of wounds will heal spontaneously. An appropriate environment is conducive to cellular healing.

Current therapeutic approaches:

1. Daily visual inspection.
2. Relieve wounds from pressure and irritation i.e. padding, pillows, protective frames, etc.
3. Frequent debridement
4. Antibiotics to control infection (intravenously, orally or locally)
5. Vasodilators to promote circulation.
6. Elevation of limbs to assist venous and lymphatic drainage
7. Frequent dressing changes
8. The application of topical antibiotic gels, lotions, etc.
9. Hyperbaric chamber (minimally utilized in most settings)

A plethora of dressings, topical agents and other antibiotics are available in the marketplace. Prolonged use however increases the risk of concomitant infections (i.e. pseudomonas) can cause an increase in pain, all are expensive and have limited benefit. Indeed recent studies indicate that topical applications as well as other medications frequently macerate cells, resulting in the inability of the wound to heal, which leads to eventual amputation. It should be quite clear that whereas some of the nursing aspects of wound healing are useful, others need revision. This will be discussed further in our approach to wound healing. In our clinic at this time, we see an increasing number of dermal ulcers in patients receiving inappropriate care. With only rare exceptions we find that all ulcers can be healed over a period varying from one week to 4 months at the extreme, if patients are cooperative and compliant.

Other impediments to healing:

- Age
- Lack of mobility
- Obesity
- Nutritional deficiencies including vitamins and minerals.
- Immune deficiency

Physiology of Wound Healing

The natural healing process can be divided into 4 phases that generally take from 6 weeks to several years.

1. **Inflammatory phase** - initiated by tissue insult; usually consists of bleeding, vasoconstriction, clot formation and the release of various chemical substances into the wound to start the healing process.
2. **Proliferative phase** - the matrix or latticework of new cells and blood vessels are laid down to provide oxygenation and a base to sustain the growth of cells and the production of proteins (collagen).
3. **Remodeling phase** - the collagen framework becomes more organized and strength of tissue increases
4. **Epithelialization** - the exterior layer of epithelial cells is completed, forming a protective barrier between the external environment and the body. This protects against fluid loss and infection.

Economics of Wound Healing

Dr. G. Woodbury et al at the University of Western Ontario have published several papers on this problem with some interesting conclusions. One study included a survey of 14,000 patients at 45 healthcare institutions and was focused on the problem of pressure ulcers. It revealed that 25% of the lesions were found in acute care hospitals, 30% in nursing homes, 22% in mixed facilities and 15% under the auspices of community care. The cost of treatment on average was found to be $24,000.00 for 12 weeks i.e. $2,000.00 per week within the healthcare facility. Cost of treatment in the community was slightly higher at $27,000.00 for a 12 week period.

- 60,000 Canadians at any time have chronic bedsores.
- 2 million Canadians have diabetes; 7.2% of these will develop ulcers of the lower extremity within the next year (150,000).
- 90,000 Canadians have spinal cord injuries and approximately 50% of these will develop pressure ulcers.

Extrapolating from these studies and relevant literature indicates that more than 250,000 Canadians have dermal ulcers at any one time. This is a conservative estimate. In North America on a pro rata basis this indicates that 3 million individuals require care for these problems on an ongoing basis and more than 60 million are afflicted on a global basis. The economic aspects of this scenario are astronomical. Resulting morbidity and mortality rates are staggering to say the least and the numbers are rising.

The Meditech Approach to Wound Healing

Over the course of the past 2 years, we have developed the following programme.

The basic platform in all conditions involves localized treatment of the ulcer site utilizing the BioFlex Laser System. This is frequently combined with therapy over the spinal nerve roots of the dermatome enervating the ulcer area peripherally. Irradiation of the autonomic nervous system along with the terminal spinal cord produces a sympathectomy type effect which significantly dilates the small arterial channels. Initially and where limbs are in jeopardy, treatment can be carried out on a daily basis for 3-4 days and can then be reduced gradually to 2-3 times per week. Geographical considerations may dictate treatment on either a daily basis or a 3 - 4 times per week schedule.

- Elevation of the limbs as much of the time as possible particularly where edema is involved.
- Protection of the ulcer by a device to prevent contact.
- Leave wound open to the atmosphere (dressings irritate, prevent moisture from escaping and reduce oxygenation).
- Treat concomitant conditions such as diabetes, lymphedema etc.
- In the early phase when devitalized tissue and bacteria are still present, cleanse gently using Q-tips soaked in hydrogen peroxide 3-4 times daily (after one week hydrogen peroxide should be diluted 100:1).
- Compress as much of the time as possible with warm saline.
- The hyperbaric chamber should be employed in critical conditions where imminent gangrene may be a factor. This is a useful adjunct and may be continued until complete healing occurs.

In order to emphasize the effectiveness of our treatment, we present 6 examples of problems that we have treated recently or are still continuing therapy.

Case Profile 1:
This patient had longstanding ulcers with osteomyelitis and was on the point of requiring amputation. Currently, the ulcers are fully healed along with the osteomyelitis and the patient is fully active.

Diagnosis:

Congenital Myopathy – 53 year old male
Chronic ulcers (2) left lower extremity and osteomyelitis with osteomyelitis metatarsal 5.
Degenerative osteoarthritis with nerve root compression left lower extremity secondary to disc herniation L4-5.

Duration of Symptoms:

Several years including long term conventional therapy i.e. antibiotics, various ointments, dressings
Amputation of 4th toe due to gangrene 3 years ago.

Treatment:

Laser, saline compresses, ulcers cleansed with hydrogen peroxide

Initial

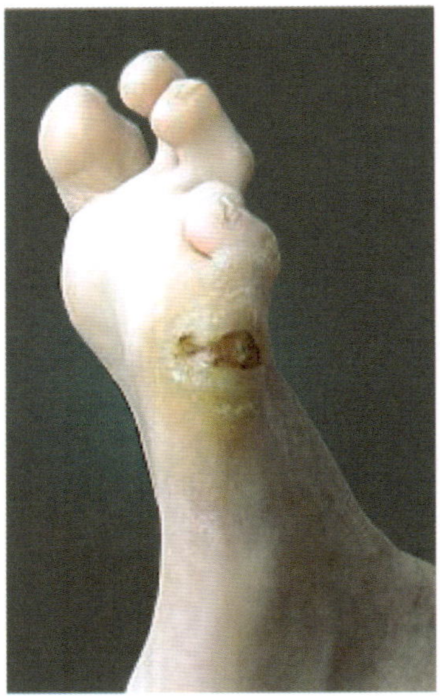

Congenital Myopathy (no sensation in lower extremities)

Interim

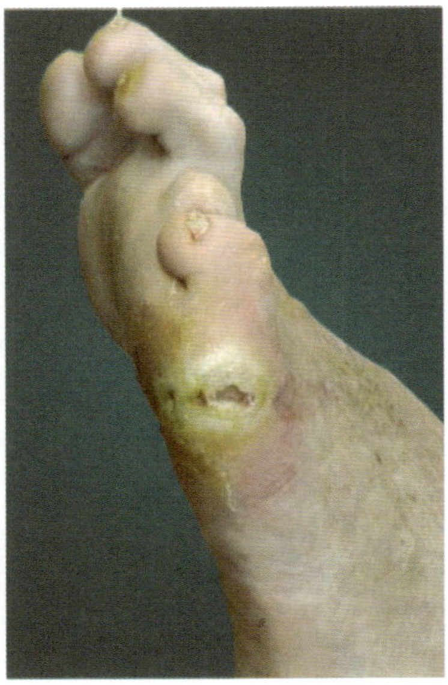

After 5 treatments

Final

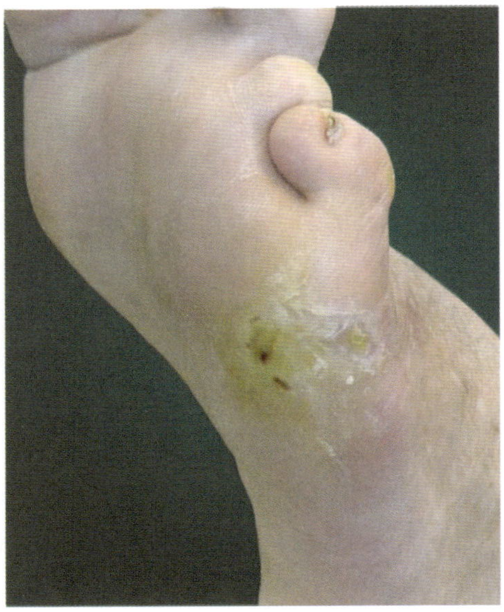

After 16 Treatments
Complete healing of ulcers (2)

Case Profile 2:
Again this demonstrates the advantage of removing dressings and initiating intensive laser therapy both locally and over the nerve roots. The patient had been on hyperbaric therapy prior to initiating laser therapy without significant improvement.

Diagnosis:

1. Diabetes.
2. Gangrene forefoot with multiple ulcers secondary to arteriosclerosis.

Duration of Symptoms:

12 months – during which patient had daily dressing changes and intensive antibiotic therapy
Amputation of left leg 3 years ago – scheduled to have right leg amputated December 4 2004.

Symptoms:

Difficulty weight bearing due to pain

Physical Findings:

- Cold, discolored and somewhat cyanotic forefoot
- Several ulcers which are not healing
- No pulses are present distal to the popliteal
- No significant venous filling in the forefoot
- The forefoot is stiff and there is no movement in the toes

Treatment:

Laser, saline compresses, ulcers cleansed with hydrogen peroxide

Initial

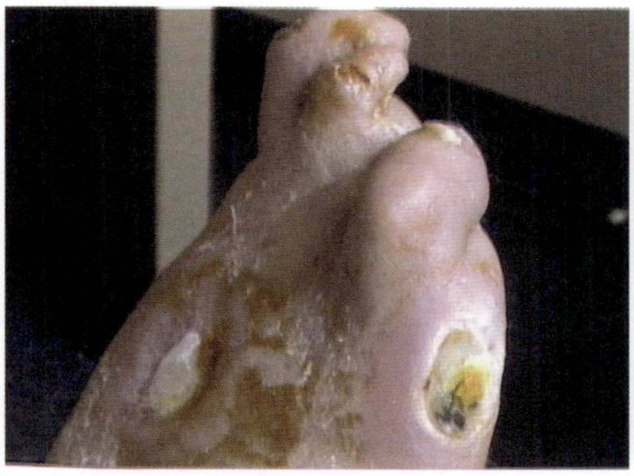

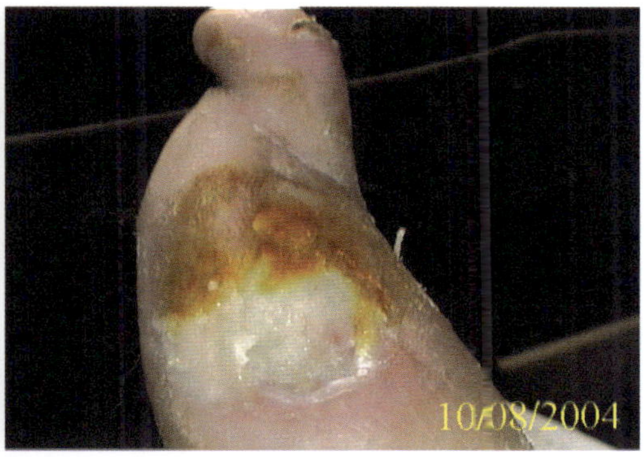

Intermediate

(After six 1-hour laser treatments)

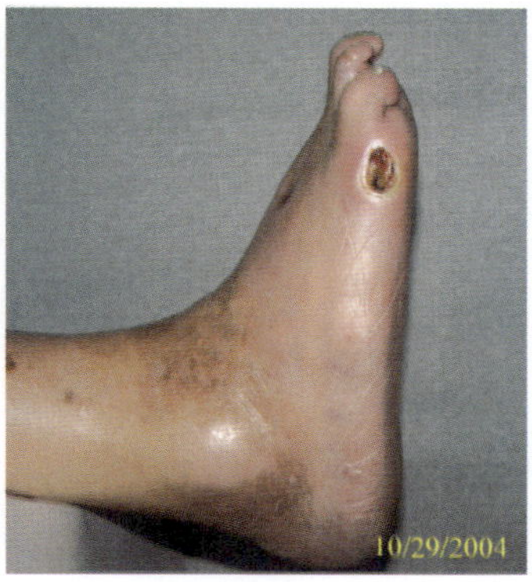

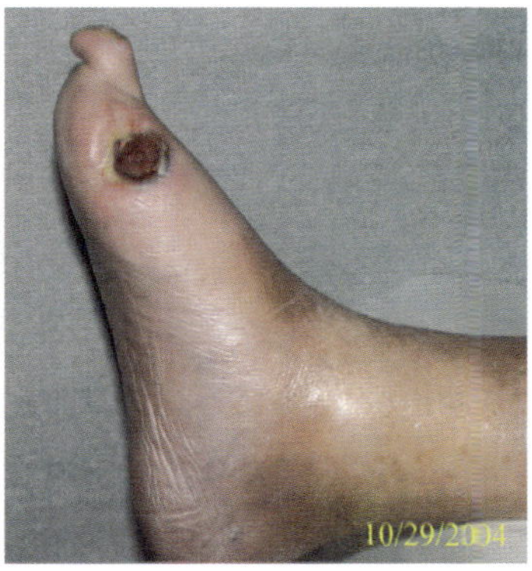

Case Profile 3:
This was a complex problem and resistant to all treatments prior to laser therapy. At this time, healing is almost complete and the thrombophlebitis has been resolved. This patient demonstrated some negative psychological aspects of these chronic/acute conditions, particularly the lack of compliance.

Diagnosis:

1. Thrombophlebitis left lower extremity.
2. Multiple Dermal Ulcers.

Duration of Symptoms:

14 months
Hospitalized December 2004 - March 2005

- Multiple biopsies with dermal breakdown
- Right calf diameter 6cm greater than left

Treatment:

Laser, saline compresses - all other medications discontinued early in course of treatment.

Initial

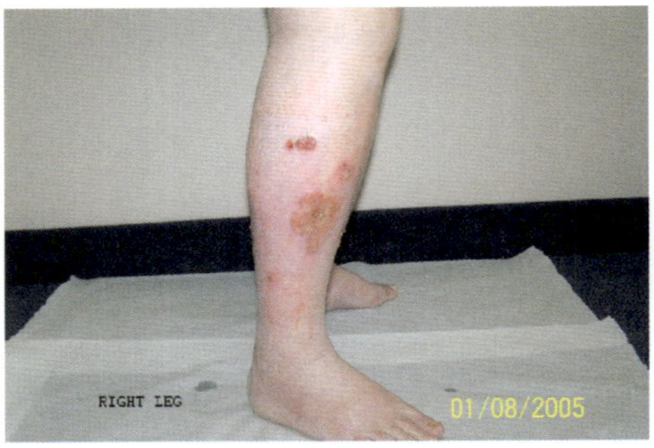

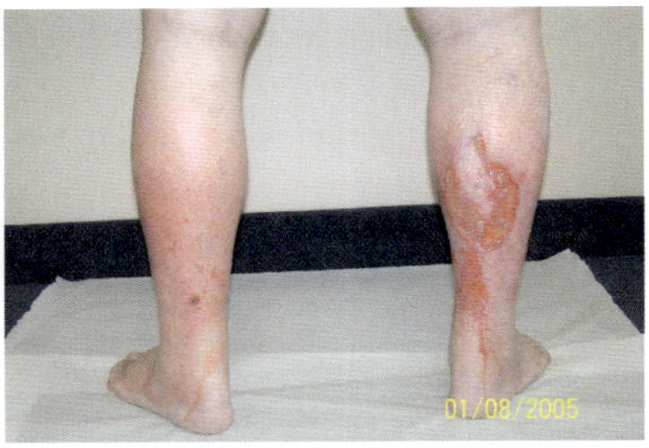

Intermediate

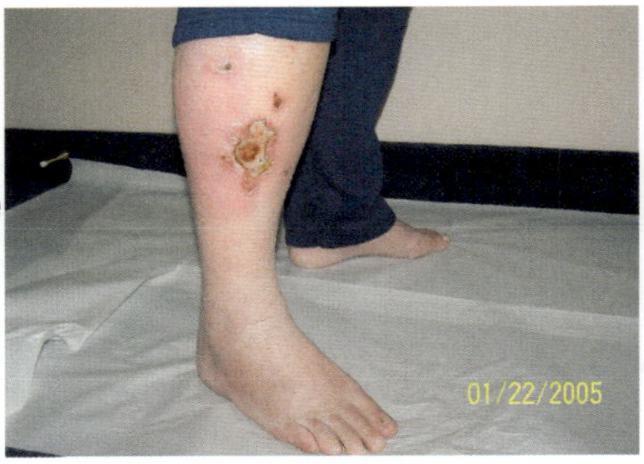

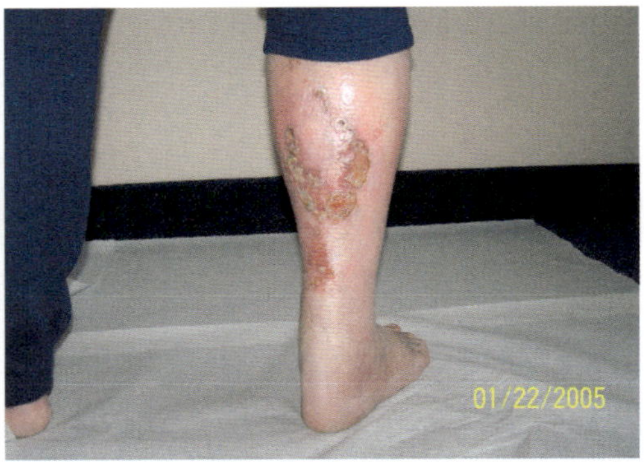

Final

- Healing almost complete

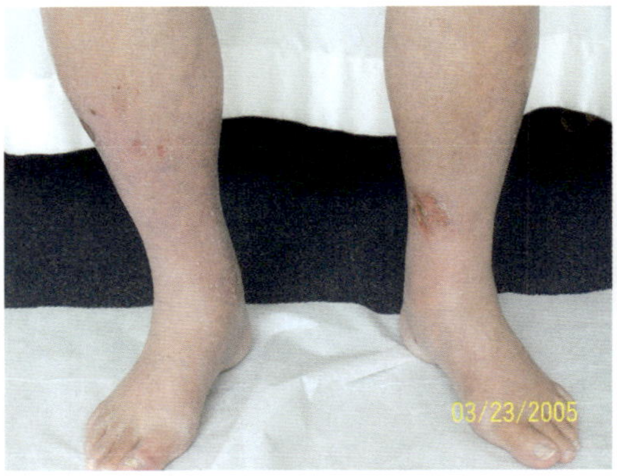

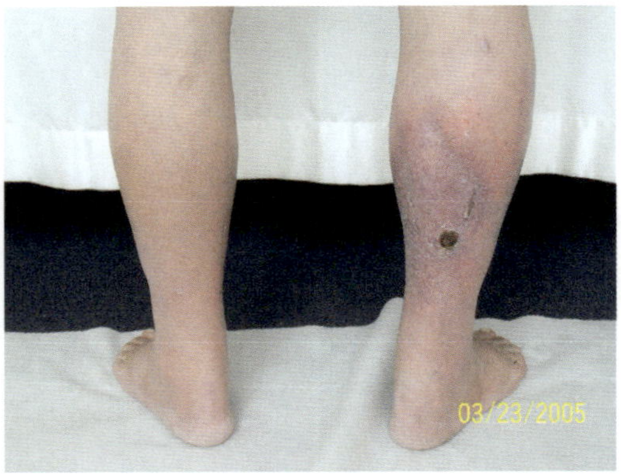

Case Profile 4:
The case demonstrates the effectiveness of wound healing using low intensity laser therapy. A 32 year old male who was in bed for several months due to severe back pain was successfully treated for degenerative osteoarthritis. With his new mobility he went for his first walk and promptly fell on his hands and elbow. Following 4 treatments using a variation of the Dermatological Protocol his wound had healed and he had regained full range of motion.

Diagnosis:

Hematoma of the left elbow
Wound of the left elbow

Duration of Symptoms:

9 days

Treatment:

Laser Therapy

Initial

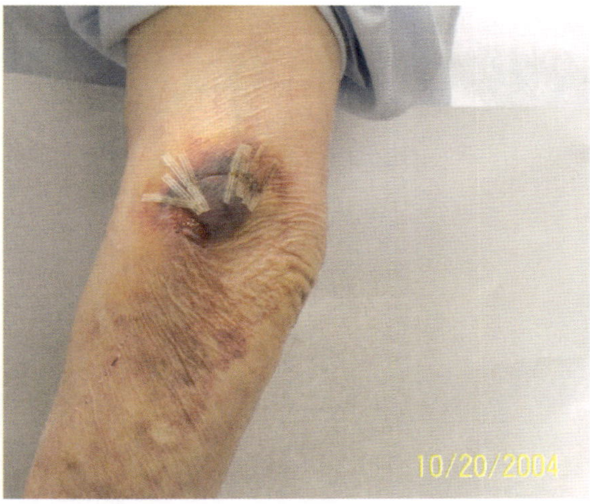

Final

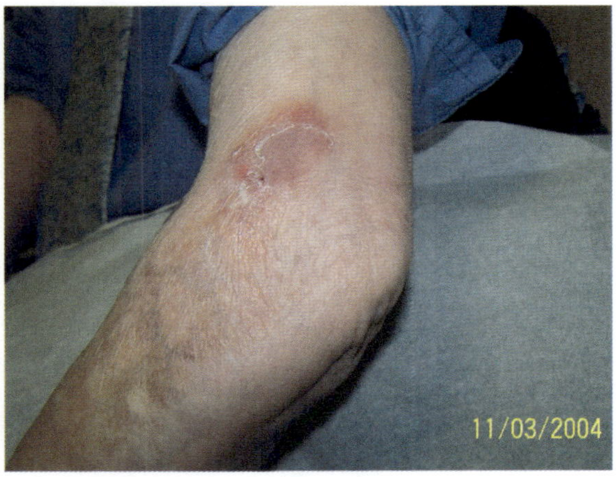

Case Profile 5:
This case demonstrates the advantages of open wound healing. Dressings and local therapies were discontinued immediately and after 5 treatments the ulcer was almost completely healed.

Diagnosis:

1. Chronic lymphedema right leg
2. Ulcer lateral aspect right ankle

Duration of Symptoms:

5 months

Surgery October 21 2004: - plate and screws, ulcer not healing
- right calf diameter 7cm greater than left

Treatment:

Laser, saline compresses - all other medications discontinued

Initial

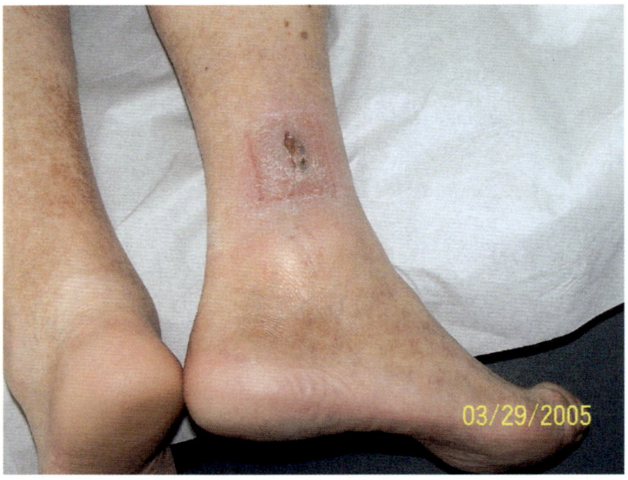

Final Picture

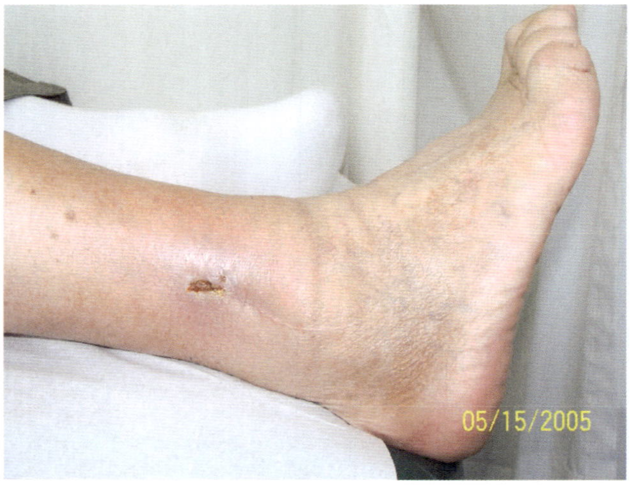

(Healing complete but patient unavailable for pitcure)

Case Profile 7:

This case demonstrates the advantages of open wound healing. Dressings, local therapies and antibiotics were discontinued on presentation and after 5 treatments the ulcers were healing rapidly. After 15 sessions the ulcers were completely epithelialized and asymptomatic.

Diagnosis:

Ulcers of the left buttock; post CVA

Duration of Symptoms:

8 months - No progression in healing with conventional methods

Treatment:

15 laser treatments over 8 weeks

Following 5 Treatments

- Infection resolved and early epithelialization

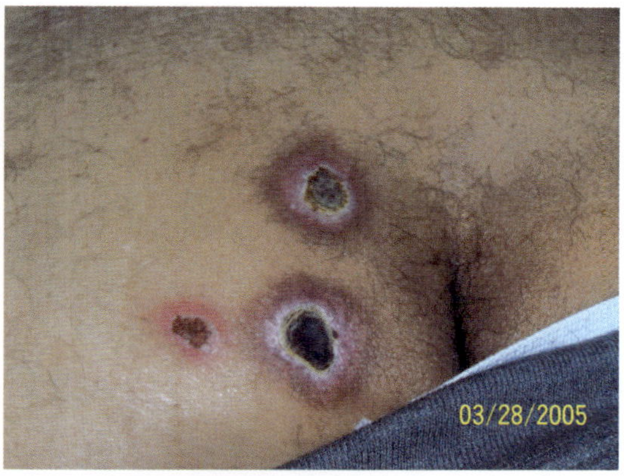

Intermediate

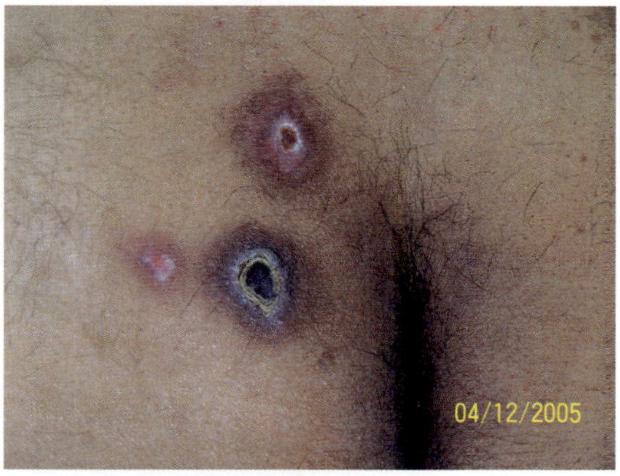

Near Final

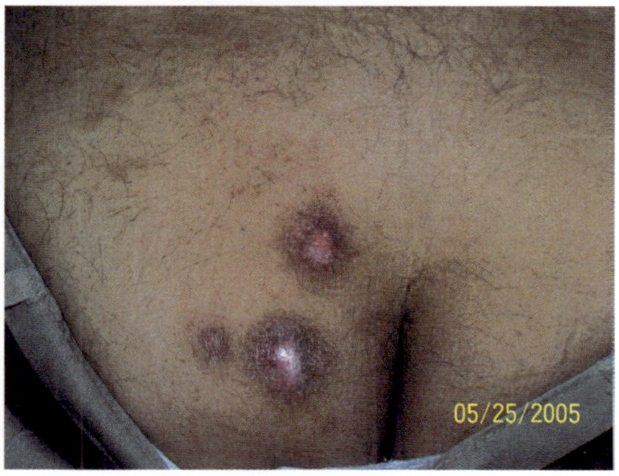

Conclusions

- The current therapeutic approach of healthcare professionals with regard to wound management must be changed.
- The teaching of wound care in medical educational institutions must be revised.
- The average cost of treating a wound/ulcer at our facility in less than $1,000.00. Compared to some of the numbers provided, this is considerably below the cost with current ineffective approaches.
- It has been stipulated that the care of a diabetic ulcer followed by amputation can be as much as $200,000.00 over a 2 year period.
- Pharmaceuticals should be avoided as much as possible as increasingly they appear to be implicated in the retardation of the healing process.
- We strongly suggest that the Meditech approach to wound healing be widely adapted in hospitals, nursing and retirement homes and the community.
- Based upon our clinical experience, most wounds may be healed by using a combination of proper systemic and environmental controls along with Low Intensity Laser Therapy as the basic platform in the healing process.
- Our experience over the past 2 years clearly indicates that Low Intensity Laser Therapy is the treatment of choice in dealing with these conditions.

The implications of the above comments are obvious. It should be apparent that particularly from the patient's welfare perspective Low Intensity Laser Therapy must be more widely applied in the treatment of all wounds and ulcers, economic factors notwithstanding.

For References, see Bibliography.

Back-Ache

November 2005

Over the millennia as man evolved from homo sapiens into homo erectus, he has been increasingly plagued by the all-inclusive term known as "back ache". Transformed over the centuries from an active hunter/farmer with a powerful musculature, based on the axiom of "survival of the fittest", the human race has become largely sedentary and in the age of technology, relatively immobile.

The result – muscle atrophy, diminished bulk, tone and flexibility; good posture is relegated to the past, and the spinal column literally collapses. This deterioration creates numerous biomechanical imbalances. The result of these developments places increasing stress on the vertebrae, discs and ligaments that form and maintain the basic infrastructure of the body.

The spine, which is the pillar of the architecture, is no longer supported by a vibrant musculature. This is comparable to the bricks and mortar around a steel skyscraper and when this breaks down it results in numerous pathological conditions which can be extremely painful and physically restrictive (Figure 1).

The inherent problems are compounded by weekend or periodic strenuous activities on the part of the individual whose tissues are dormant during the week and are then subjected to physical stress for which they are not prepared. The recommended "minutes" of stretching prior to activity is really of minimal help. This is one of the major mobility problems facing bipeds in the age of technology. As people live longer, tissues are also subjected to the "wear and tear" of the aging process, characterized as "degenerative osteoarthritis". The combination of disuse due to the sedentary factor and degeneration of the tissues as a result of aging, produces multiple problems of the joints, cartilage and soft tissues of the spine, for reasons which are readily apparent. The spine supports the weight of the upper body and the functional stress imposed by the lower body and by virtue of its perpendicular state the complexity of the discs, vertebrae, facets, etc. make it the largest and certainly the most vulnerable structure in the entire body.

As degeneration progresses there is increasing osteophyte formation, chronic and acute inflammation of the surrounding tissues, scar tissue formation, joint contracture, etc. Other more ominous complications accompany these events (i.e. stenosis, a narrowing of the spinal canal with compression of the cord and the foramina through which nerve roots exit from the spinal canal).

In high level athletes the process is dramatically accelerated. Excessive exposure to high levels of activity speeds up the wear and tear phenomenon. It is not unusual in our practice to see fifteen year old gymnasts with spinal X-rays and symptoms that resemble someone in the 6th or 7th decade of life; a rather elementary conclusion one might add. Whether secondary to activity, trauma or degeneration, back-ache has become one of the major healthcare problems in our society and the economic impact is astronomical.

Few individuals go through life without back problems and the burden on the healthcare system increases exponentially as people live longer and increasingly develop arthritis. The elderly whose problems all too frequently are neglected, often end up in a wheelchair; the younger and healthier members of society following traumatic episodes lapse into a lifetime of inactivity. Both add to the socio-economic burden.

Back problems are seldom simple and often complex. Even a routine disc herniation occurring in a teenager while sneezing during a moment of relaxation of the musculature, results in nerve root compression and scar tissue formation. Chemicals released from the disintegration of the nucleosus pulposus may cause acute/chronic irritation of nerve roots much as osteophytes, disc fragments and scar tissue result in nerve root compression, often with loss of sensation or even motor paralysis.

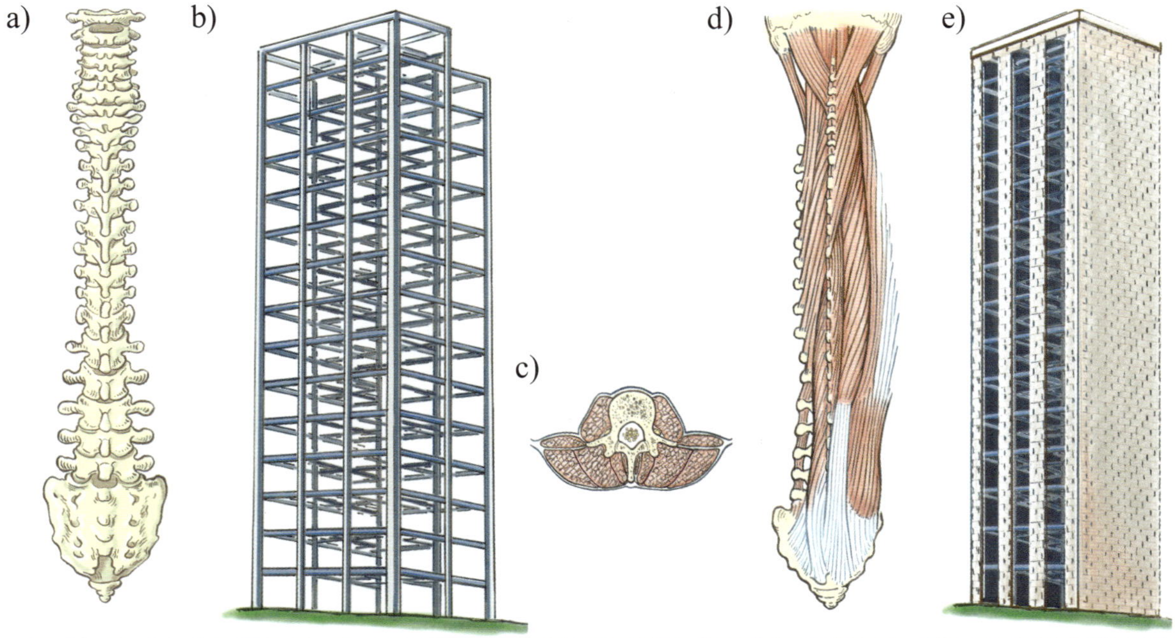

Figure 8	a) Spinal column without support is extremely vulnerable to force and stress.	b) Steel infrastructure of a skyscraper without bricks and mortar would collapse with minimal stress.	c) Cross section of spine with musculature. (Muscles comprise 75-80% of the bulk)	d) Spinal column with muscle is 5 times more resistant to force and stress than bone alone.	e) Building with concrete and mortar has a much greater stress tolerance than steel alone.

Maintenance and Prevention

Muscle strengthening, stretching and maintenance programmes based on exercise are helpful. In the advancing years, these should be moderate in degree but daily and vigorous; generally one half hour plus in duration (i.e. stretching, swimming, walking, Pilates, Yoga, etc.). This will keep the muscles strong and the tissues flexible. For optimum health this measure should be complemented with a balanced diet, vitamin and mineral supplements and the avoidance of inappropriate stress both physical and mental.

If the above methodologies are instituted in a disciplined, systematic fashion, most pathological conditions are minimized, delayed or avoided completely. Once symptoms have become established and cannot be controlled by conventional measures (i.e. analgesics, anti-inflammatories (NSAIDS), muscle relaxants and cortisone) a serious problem develops. The aforementioned measures simply mask or modulate symptoms but have no healing effect on the cells which compose the various tissue structures.

In due course, surgery may be necessary (i.e. joint replacements, laminectomy, discectomies, fusions, etc.). In essence these therapies have limited curative benefit with regard to cellular health and indeed in most cases produce a long term deleterious effect that may be more harmful than the original disease.

All conventional therapies currently in use modulate symptoms but do not cure the pathology. Surgery attempts to repair the problem and is sometimes successful, but more frequently than not it falls short of its objectives and may make the condition worse and irreversible.

Factors Contributing to Back Problems

1) Lack of exercise accompanied by loss of muscle mass, tone and flexibility
2) Dietary imbalances, depriving tissues of the proteins necessary to maintain muscle bulk
3) Depletion of hormone production (i.e. H.G.F. Estrogen, Testosterone)
   - concomitant with aging, systemic diseases, etc.
4) Obesity which further increases the stress factor of the spinal column
5) High level sports accelerating the wear and tear process
6) Vehicular accidents resulting in STI, fractures, whiplash type injuries, etc.

Table 16. Classification of Therapies:

Symptom Modulation:	Definitive Therapies:
- Analgesics & NSAIDs	- Surgery
- Muscle relaxants	- Laser
- Cortisone	
- Interferential Current	
- Ultrasound	
- Diathermy/ Ice	
- Manipulation	
- Massage (shiatsu, swedish, etc.)	

Economic Impact of Back Ache/Pain

Statistics (U.S. Based):

- 90% of all individuals experience severe pain at some point in their life
- 26 million adults in the US suffer from back ache (10% of the population at any one time)
- 5 million Americans are permanently disabled in varying degrees by back pain
- 2 million Americans cannot work as a result of back problems
- Low back pain is responsible for close to a hundred million work-days lost per annum
- The economic loss is over 5 billion in healthcare dollars on an annualized basis
- Pain secondary to arthritis affects 40 million Americans and results in over 4 billion dollars in lost income per annum
- Close to 50 million Americans suffer chronic recurrent headaches resulting from back problems and spend close to 5 billion dollars a year on a variety of medications. The toxic effects of the numerous medications are incalculable (i.e. hepatic failure, renal failure, gastrointestinal bleeding, etc.) This seriously impacts patient health.

Pathological Conditions

1) Myofascitis (inflammation of overlying muscles and fascia, adhesions, scar tissue)
2) Herniated/bulging discs (Figure 10)
3) Degenerative disc disease (D.D.D.) (Figure 9)
4) Scar tissue contractures
5) Osteophyte formation (Figure 9)
6) Stenosis - foramina, spinal canal (Figure 9,11&13)
7) SI joint dysfunction
8) Facet joint syndrome (Figure 13)

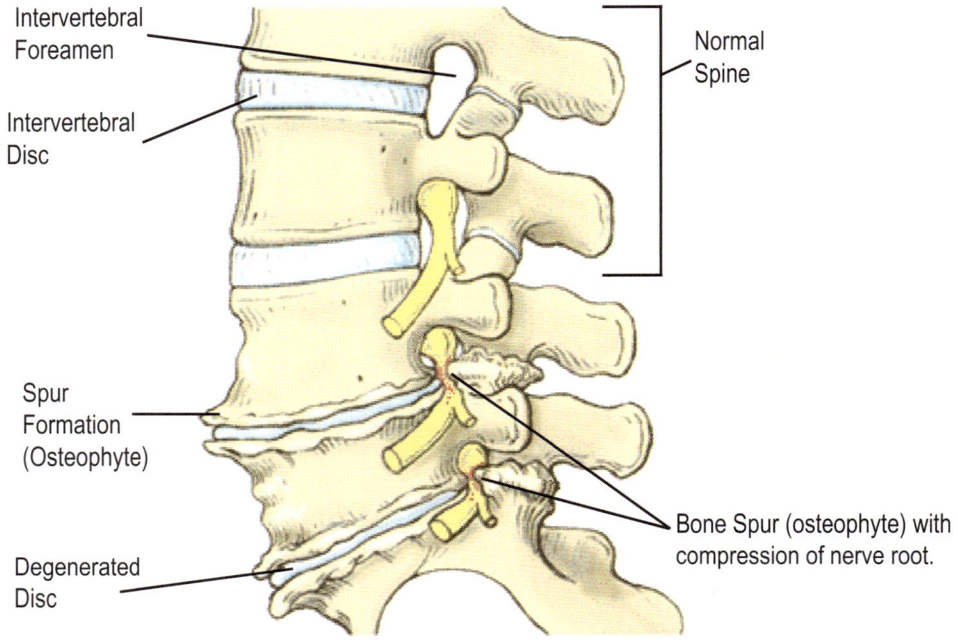

Figure 9. Degenerative Disc Disease resulting in compression of the spinal nerve roots.

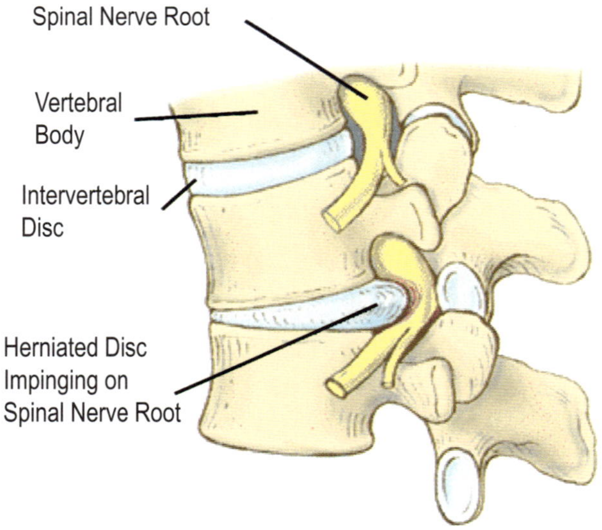

Figure 10. A diagram of a single disc herniation with compression of nerve root (usually in younger age groups).

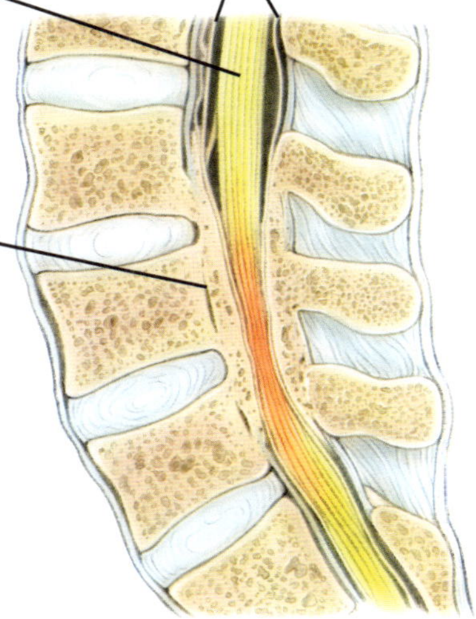

Figure 11. A diagram of spinal stenosis resulting from osteophyte formation.

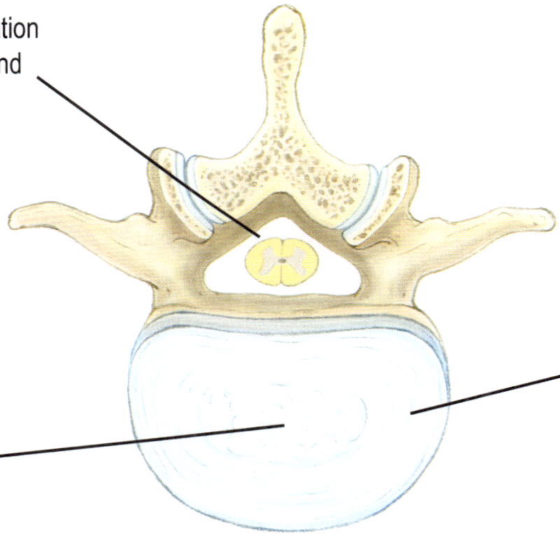

Figure 12. Normal spinal canal with ample space for spinal cord.

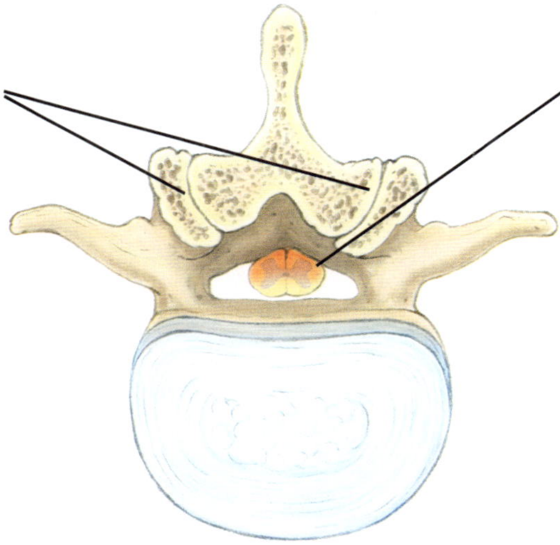

Figure 13. Spinal stenosis (lacking adequate space for spinal cord transit).

Conclusions

Probably the greatest beneficiaries of our technology are individuals that suffer from back pain and arthritis. This includes athletes suffering from myofascitis, facet joint syndrome, sacroiliac joint dysfunction and disc herniations with nerve root compression. More significantly, dramatic effects are obtained by sufferers of chronic degenerative osteoarthritis accompanied by spinal/foraminal stenosis with attendant neurological complications.

Many of the patients who come to us, either through word of mouth or referred by healthcare providers, arrive in wheelchairs or utilize canes; many have been bedridden for years. Usually after five to twenty treatments which are totally noninvasive, painless and easily applied, they become ambulatory and voluntarily lose their drug dependencies along with their mechanical supports. More significantly they experience the elimination of pain and regain mobility and quality of life.

Included are patients who have been taking up to thirty Tylenol tablets per day and over the past years have taken as many as fourteen medications at the same time. The latter in itself often results in addiction problems, sometimes worse than the basic pathology.

The most promising and least known technology currently available and one that can be delivered in a highly scientific non-invasive fashion is Low Intensity Laser Therapy. Unfortunately most patients and therapists including MDs, chiropractors, physiotherapists, etc. have little knowledge or awareness of this approach, and in the economic climate today, have little interest in exploring new technologies that are superior, but are not included in the "spider web" of compensatory codes imposed by HMO's, insurance companies and governments.

At Meditech we have developed a delivery system that is currently the most advanced on a global basis achieving a significant improvement/cure rate with all the above entities. Low Intensity Laser Therapy is truly the ideal therapeutic approach for back problems in the 21st century.

The therapy acts by converting light into biochemical energy, resulting in normal cell morphology and function, which causes symptoms to disappear. Aside from the gradual elimination of inflammation, various degrees of the ablation of scar tissue, and osteophytes at all levels, there appears to be little question that a thin layer of cartilaginous regeneration can occur. In our teaching clinic, attached to our corporate headquarters, we perform 600 patient treatments weekly and our significant improvement/cure rate is in excess of 93 percent.

Patients at the completion of the treatment often state "Why doesn't my doctor know about this?" As Marshall McLuhan said, "The medium is the message." Perhaps the medium should re-evaluate its objectives.

With "back problems" laser therapy should be the universal treatment approach and clearly establish its role as the treatment of choice. Thousands of our patients would agree.

Herpes Zoster (Shingles): A Therapy at Last

November 2005

Low Intensity Laser Therapy when properly applied has an infinite ability to heal. Along with a number of systemic, dermatological and musculoskeletal problems, we may be able to now add shingles to the list of conditions where Low Intensity Laser Therapy may be applied as an effective therapy.

Over the past two years at our rehabilitation centre, we have treated a number of patients afflicted with this sometimes severe viral infection and have been universally successful in treating these conditions.

Herpes in its many forms has long defied traditional therapeutic solutions; at present these comprise:

- Analgesics for pain.
- Anti-inflammatories to reduce the edema/erythema.
- Antivirals to reduce viral replication and shedding.
- Antibiotics to treat secondary bacterial infections.
- A variety of topical ointments.
- Cortisone in severe cases

In essence, there is no definitive approach and the therapies listed above simply modulate symptoms at best.

Symptoms:

- patient feels unwell (prodromal phase - may last from one day to two weeks)
- rash consisting of red spots followed by blister formation
- area extremely sensitive to touch and contact of any kind
- localized to one side of body only and follows nerves (dermatomes)
- may heal by scarring
- pain may be prolonged, along with extreme fatigue and other symptomatology concomitant with the disease

Course:

- must have previous history of chickenpox
- outbreaks are generally related to stress, immune suppression, infections, tumors and the use of pharmaceuticals

Pathogenesis:

Etiological factor is the varicella-zoster virus. Following an outbreak of chickenpox the virus lies dormant within the cells and neural pathways for many years after the patient has had the original attack.

- virus reactivates under the stimulus of stressful conditions
- may cause facial paralysis, blindness, encephalitis
- virus is present at site of rash and is contagious for up to a week after blisters develop
- more common in elderly but younger age groups not excluded

A vexing complication is post herpetic neuralgia as these patients continue to suffer from the signs and symptoms despite treatment with conventional therapies. The pain is not relieved and can be excruciating along with multiple serious sequelae.

There is some evidence that acyclovir and other antiviral drugs slow reproduction of the virus in the nerve cells but this is effective only to varying degrees and is not curative.

In the US, over one million people develop shingles annually and a significant percentage of these develop a complication called post herpetic neuralgia. The pain in these individuals may persist for months and years. The characteristics of this infection vary, are resistant to all forms of treatment and are prolonged. This can lead to depression and a total inability to function.

A number of treatments have been applied for this condition:

- Lidoderm
- Tens
- Nerve blocks
- Epidural injections

Again, these therapeutic approaches attempt to alter symptoms but do not cure the problem. A vaccine developed in 1995, is useful in prevention but has not been widely utilized. This vacine only has a 20 year effective duration. If children are innoculated early in life it leaves them prone to the more dangerous form of disease later in life, whereas being infected with chickenpox leaves them virtually immune for life.

The virus lodges in nerve pathways, myelin sheaths and cells. As the photos indicate we have treated a significant number of these type of problems over the past 2 years, with a rapid curative effect particularly in dealing with the post herpetic neuralgia problem. Post herpetic neuralgia generally persists long after the dermal lesions have disappeared, therefore cannot be pictorially displayed. It is suggested that low intensity laser therapy is the treatment of choice in these situations.

Herpes Simplex

Often, we see other herpes type lesions caused by viruses belonging to the same family of organisms i.e. herpes labialis (cold sores), herpes genitalis (lesions of the genito-urinary tract), etc. that are all variations of Herpes Simplex.

Presented here is a brief discussion of Herpes Simplex, the most common form of herpes. It has an overall prevalence of 20% in the United States, with a slightly higher proportion of infected females (26%) than males (18%). These cases are much easier to treat and resolve. Inevitably they will resolve spontaneously over the course of time.

There are two main benefits of Low Intensity Laser Therapy in treating Herpes Simplex. The first is the rapid resolution of symptoms such as edema, blisters, pain, etc. This effect is most likely due to a number of physiological processes (i.e. increased micro vascular perfusion, improved cellular metabolism, etc.). The second benefit is a reduction in future outbreaks following treatment with LILT. A double blind clinical trial on the effects of LILT on herpes simplex (Shindl & Neumann, 1999) reported that after 10 treatments with LILT the average reoccurence-free interval between outbreaks was 37.5 weeks, compared to 3 weeks in the placebo group. The results of this study support the clinical experience at Meditech, proving that following treatment with LILT the symptoms are resolved more rapidly and symptom free periods are of longer duration.

Inital **Intermediate**

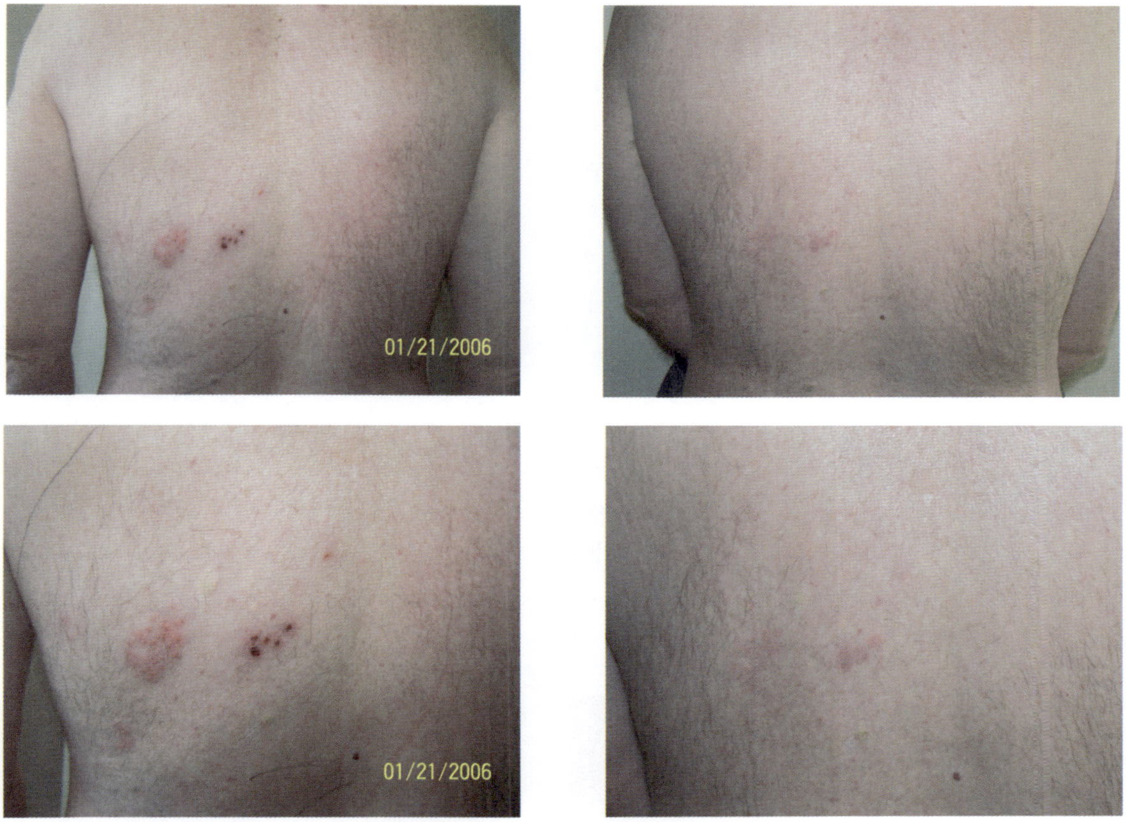

Patient 1. Male 57 years;
Acute episode of Shingles and post herpetic neuralgia.
4 treatments over 8 days. Asymptomatic

Initial

Final

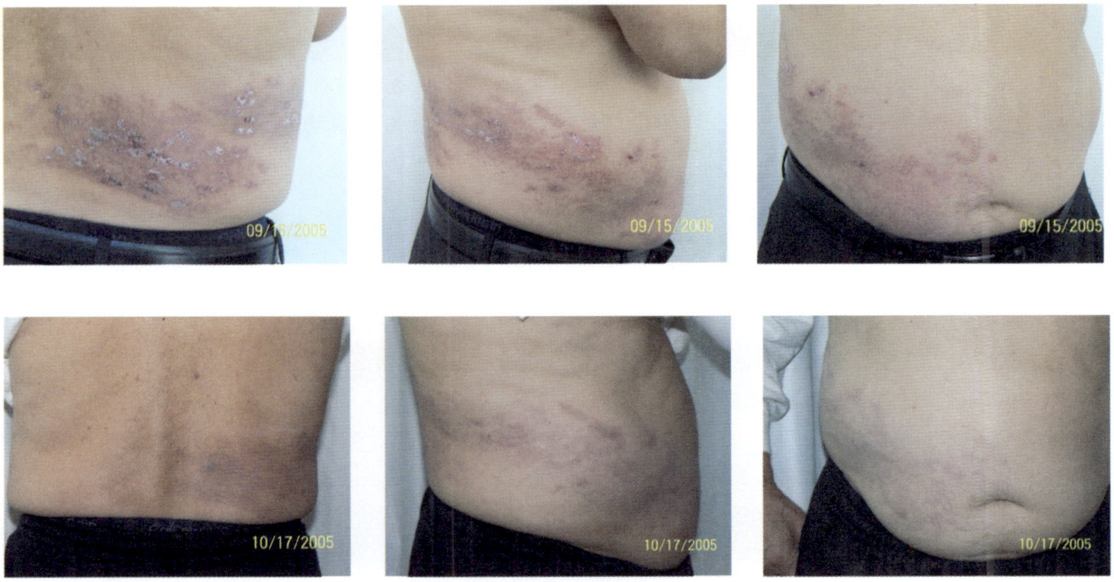

Patient 2. Male 72 years;
Acute episode of Shingles and post herpetic neuralgia.
8 treatments over 1 month. (First visit 6 weeks post onset of initial symptoms)

Initial Final

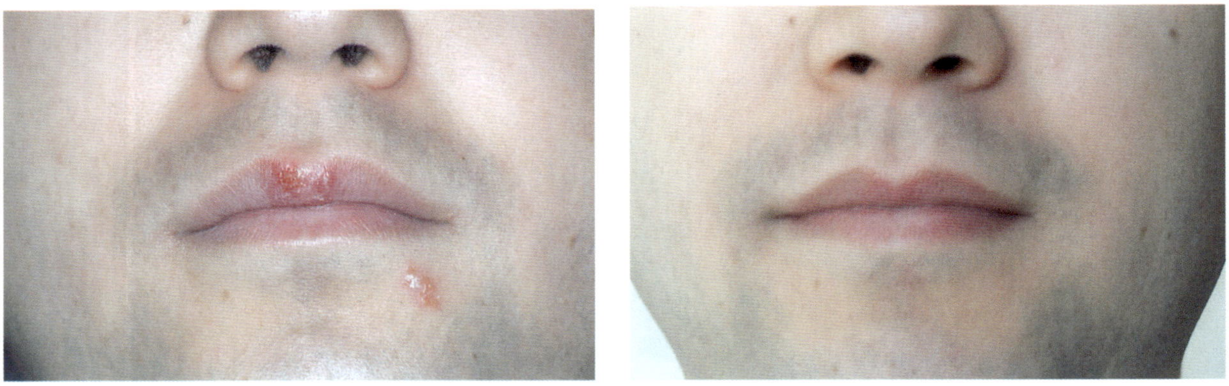

Patient 3. Male 33 years;
Acute episode of Herpes Simplex.
3 treatments over 20 days

Initial Final

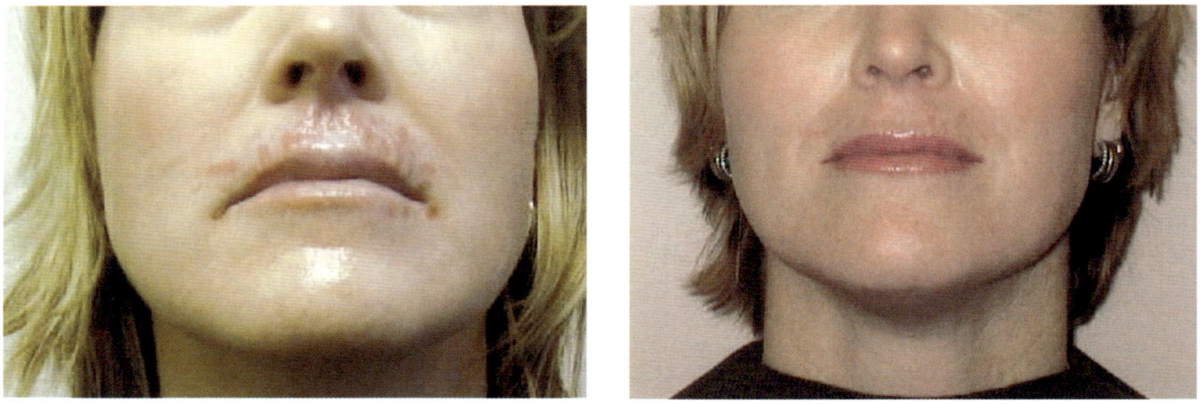

Patient 4. Female 38 years;
Acute episode of Herpes Simplex.
2 treatments over 3 days

Conclusion

Again it would be useful to perform a double blind clinical study using LILT to confirm the clinical results presented. At the same time the assumption may be made that LILT offers a safe effective solution in the treatment of a wide range of viral infections.

The previous cases presented illustrate the curative effects of LILT for the treatment of Herpes Zoster (Patient 1 and Patient 2) and Herpes Simplex (Patient 3 and Patient 4).

Low Intensity Laser Therapy - Myths and Realities

February 2005

Frequently, we are asked to compare Low Intensity Laser Therapy Systems with regard to power, frequency and other parameters. Accordingly, we are hereby attempting to inform readers about the significance of these factors.

Aside from this one, should always keep in mind that the most important objective of all therapies are:

- To provide maximum clinical benefit in the shortest possible period of time.
- To do no harm to the patient.

The BioFlex Low Intensity Laser Therapy System has several proprietary features particular to its unique design which cannot be revealed for purposes of patent protection. Nevertheless, it should be understood that its flexible treatment arrays, the ability to modulate output over an infinite range and total accuracy are critical to an effective, efficient delivery system. The ability to customize treatment for any individual patient is also essential.

Discussion of the following criteria should assist in the clarification of many issues. The principals at Meditech hope that the reader will be enlightened by these explanations.

1. Myth: Higher powered devices mean better therapy.

Reality: Power is not the only factor for effective treatment using laser therapy. Other important parameters are: frequency, duty cycle, waveform, treatment duration and of course energy density (J/cm2).

2. Myth: LEDs (Light Emitting Diodes) or SLDs (Super Luminous Diodes) are not effective.

Reality: The differences between the characteristics of lasers and SLDs are:

- Lasers are monochromatic, producing light output at a single wavelength. In contrast, SLDs output a band of wavelengths. The band of wavelengths is the spectral width of the device.
- Lasers are coherent. Basically, coherence is defined as the light waves being in phase.
- Lasers are highly directional and can be easily focused to a point. In other words, lasers are less divergent than other light sources.

The higher power ratings of lasers are not obtainable with SLDs. However, the properties of lasers do not make a significant impact on the therapy when compared to SLDs for the purpose of irradiating cellular pathologies in an appropriate manner.

Wavelength(s) of the Light Source: A bandwidth that starts at approximately 600nm and ends at approximately 900nm (red-to-NIR region) has been identified as containing the wavelengths appropriate for laser therapy. No adverse effects have been documented for any wavelengths over this range. Therefore, even though SLDs emit most of their power at the rated wavelength, the additional wavelengths emitted are also a beneficial part of the therapy.

Coherence: Specially designed experiments at the cellular level have provided evidence that coherent and noncoherent light with the same wavelength, intensity, and irradiation time create equivalent biological effects. This is further supported with successful studies where SLDs were the only light sources.

Divergence: Since SLD light sources diverge more than laser sources, the SLD source spreads the light over a broader treatment area. However, the SLD would only require additional treatment time to match the dosage for an area treated by the laser source. Therefore, the energy delivered to an area can be equally produced by a SLD or a laser source with duration being the only variant.

3. Myth: Only certain wavelengths are effective.

Reality: Through many clinical trials and studies it has been documented that a range of wavelengths that starts at approximately 600nm and ends at approximately 900nm (red-to-NIR region) has been identified as the wavelengths appropriate for laser therapy to produce positive tissue response.

4. Myth: Frequency and duty cycle do not make a difference.

Reality: Clinical trials and basic research studies have revealed the importance of frequency and duty cycle with regard to treatment outcome. The ability to vary these over a wide range is essential.

5. Myth: Flexibility and contact are not important.

Reality: The power of the light decreases with the distance from the source and also attenuates as it passes through different media due to refraction and reflection. Applying the light source as close as possible to the injury produces the most effective energy transfer and therefore, the best results.

6. Myth: One protocol can be used to heal many ailments.

Reality: Clinical experience reveals that different medical conditions respond better to certain protocols than others; in addition, each individual is genetically different, therefore the ability to customize protocols is required for proper treatment.

7. Myth: Laser therapy simply modulates the symptoms and does not heal.

Reality: Light is absorbed by a variety of cellular components including chromophores, flavoproteins and other micromolecules in the tissue being irradiated. In essence, light energy is transformed into biochemical energy resulting in the restoration of normal cellular function. All tissue consists of cells and all cells respond to LILT in varying degrees.

8. Myth: All laser therapy does is heat the area being treated.

Reality: The primary healing mechanism is caused by the interaction of the light with tissue causing a number of physiological reactions. Although all light sources generate some heat, a properly designed laser therapy system minimizes the temperature rise of the treated area. Inadequately engineered devices may overheat the tissue, a substantially undesirable feature.

9. Myth: High power pulsed devices are more effective than others.

Reality: Some manufacturer's instruments pulse light at very high power and for extremely brief duration. There is no evidence that this method produces actual improvement or any significant clinical effect in cells.

10. Myth: Frequency controls depth of penetration.

Reality: The wavelength of the light is one factor that controls the depth of penetration. This myth is the result of confusion between the rate of repetition (frequency) of the applied waveform and the wavelength of the light (frequency of light equals the inverse of wavelength). The power of the light source also affects the penetration depth.

11. Myth: Shorter treatment times at higher power are better than lower power for a longer treatment period in order to reduce therapy time.

Reality: There is an overdose range at which too much power inhibits recovery of the cell and therefore the cure of the pathology being treated. One cannot concentrate power into too short a time interval in order to reduce treatment times. Tissue has physiologic limitations resulting in a prolonged period of recovery if inappropriate therapy is utilized.

12. Myth: Place many different diodes with varying wavelengths into the same treatment head for efficient use of treatment time!

Reality: Basic researchers have shown that tissue processes light stimulation more efficiently utilizing diodes of similar wavelength at any one time. Indeed it has been noted that combining diodes of different wavelengths is contraindicated if effective therapy is to be achieved.

13. Myth: Laser therapy stimulates cancer development or variants of cancer cells.

Reality: In our experience there is no evidence that shows that laser light, either causes cancer or stimulates cancer cells to divide. Indeed, with correct usage of laser light patients with metastases suffering from severe pain, pleural effusions and other complications have responded extremely well with regard to pain reduction and other problems associated with malignancies. At the same time more research is essential in order to formulate permanent conclusions in the field of cancer treatment using laser. This is an area that must be explored.

14. Myth: Laser Therapy damages tissues.

Reality: High powered devices can definitely denature protein and damage molecules. Laser therapy is only effective if used in an appropriate, clinically effective time-tested fashion.

For References, see Bibliography.

II Prescriptions

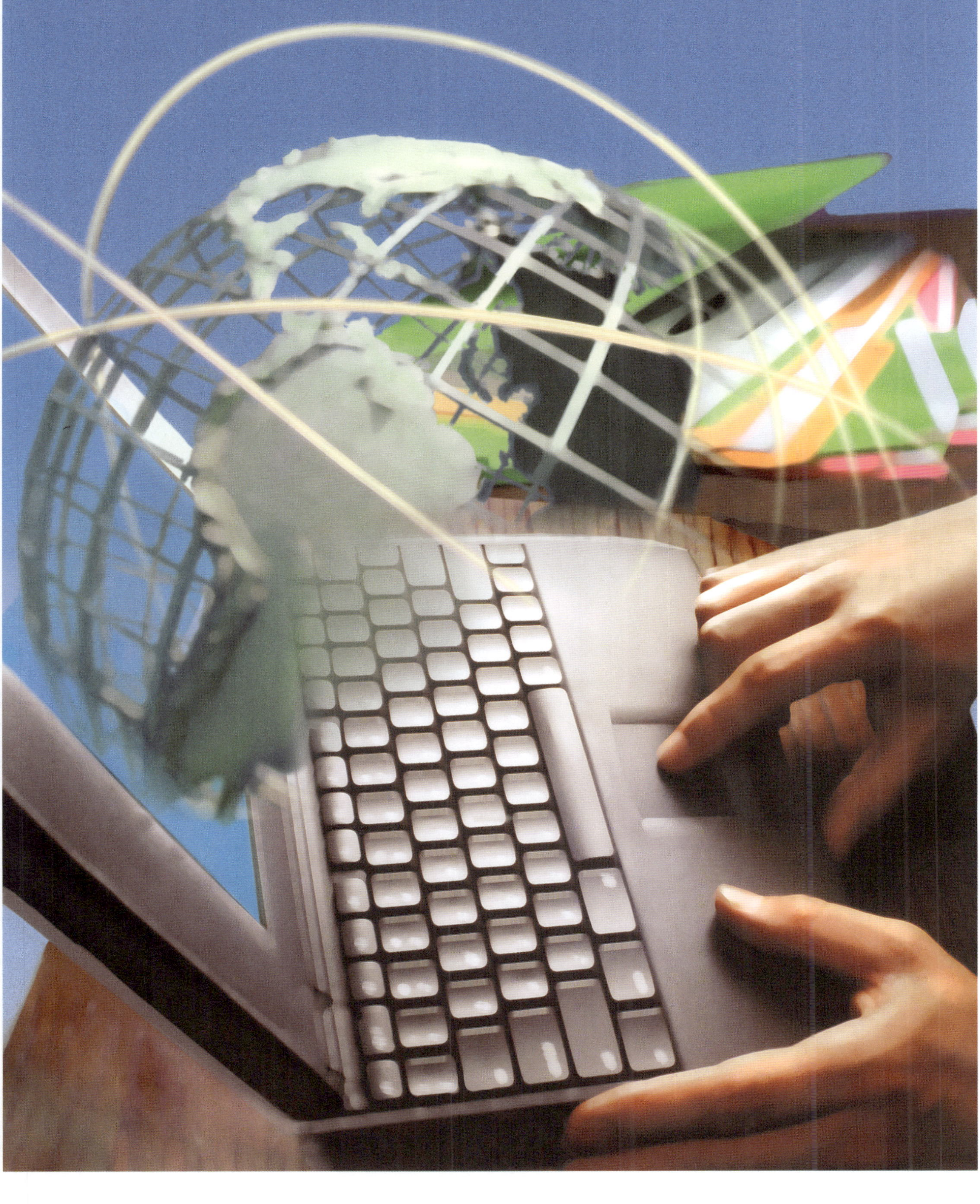

Introduction

Introduction

As a company we value our clients and the customer service that we provide. Accordingly, at this time we are pleased to bring you an update from our original protocols developed over 10 years ago. Monumental progress has been made since that time and this trend will continue; it is the focus of our technological and clinical approach.

This publication is based on 16 years of scientific research and extensive clinical experience, (over 1 million patients treated to date) with the continuing refinement of the protocols being the major objective. We also support the development of protocols by independent therapists, utilizing over 300 BioFlex Systems in 20 different countries. The BioFlex System is not only an advanced therapeutic delivery system but can also be utilized to do clinical reseach on an individual basis.

The BioFlex Therapist System is to be used only by trained health care professionals as part of a comprehensive treatment plan.

The protocols provided are highly effective in over 75% of cases; however, there is always room for further improvement. The tremendous flexibility of the BioFlex system allows therapists to safely explore the use of multiple frequencies, different waveforms and energy densities with any of the six treatment arrays available. Indeed, it is an open system with therapeutic innovation as the norm. In our corporate clinic, we compile safe new protocols on a daily basis and monitor the individuality of each patient's response. Most importantly, the utilization of these protocols will further enhance clinical effectiveness in the remaining 25% of cases. The BioFlex Therapist System should not be used during the first trimester of pregnancy.

If you require additional protocols or wish to share dramatic new protocols you may have discovered, please contact us at 416-251-1055 or info@bioflexlaser.com.

Preamble

1. On occasion, pain may increase after the first or second treatment. If that is the case, patients having been forewarned, are advised to utilize ice and analgesics. On subsequent visits, frequencies and duty cycles of all probes are appropriately reduced. For example, if the original infrared setting is 20 Hz and 40% duty cycle, these should be reduced to a frequency of 5-10 Hz and a duty cycle of 20%. On subsequent visits, they can be gradually elevated as tissue tolerance increases.
   The same rule should be observed initially in the treatment of autoimmune cases, older patients and children. In all these situations, it can be observed that as tissue tolerance develops, both frequencies and duty cycles can be increased using clinical reassessment as the appropriate guideline.
2. One should also alert patients that if the treatment array should become too warm they should advise the attendant. If an elderly patient leans back against the array placed on the spine for instance, there may be a lack of ventilation and over heating can occur. It is important to avoid using treatment heads between patients until the heads have cooled to an adequate degree. These are common sense matters but must always be observed. The therapeutic array is designed to be athermal and in order for heat to be dissipated away from the tissues, it must be properly ventilated.
3. If initial protocols are improving the condition being treated, continue to utilize these until symptoms plateau and then move to the next stage. i.e. stage 2, stage 3, etc.

Frequency of Treatment

1. In acute conditions, it may be appropriate to treat patients on a daily basis for 3-4 days. Evaluate clinically on each visit, until symptoms subside. This approach is particularly applicable in cases of trauma, herniated discs and acute back problems.
2. Once the patient is reasonably comfortable, treat three times per week until stable, then reduce to twice per week until improvement is at least 80% or more.
3. Weekly maintenance therapy may be required with degenerative osteoarthritis for two to three months or even longer in certain situations. Appropriate clinical judgement must dictate the need for continuing therapy.
4. Longer treatment sessions in many situations result in a reduced number of patient visits for each condition treated.
5. Completion of treatment in acute conditions, generally requires one to three weeks. In chronic situations such as degenerative osteoarthritis, one to two months may be required. In degenerative osteoarthritis of the lumbosacral spine with stenosis of the spinal canal and/or the foramina, up to 50 treatments may be necessary over a protracted period of time.

Discharge of Patient from Treatment Program

Discharge is appropriate when the following criteria are met.

- Relatively asymptomatic
- Fully functional
- No medications required
- Quality of life returns to normal

This period may require from one to thirty treatments.

Length of Individual Treatments

Until two years ago, we generally confined our treatment sessions to less than 40 minutes. Currently our standard treatment for most conditions is between 20 and 30 minutes, however, for back problems and pathological conditions of greater scope and depth, up to one hour may be utilized. In situations with multiple conditions, an hour may be devoted to the spine and 30 minutes to an extremity. No adverse effects have been incurred with prolonged treatment sessions. If time is a factor, treatments can be reduced to 15-20 minutes in simple localized lesions (ie. epicondylitis). Always treat the most severe problem most aggressively.

Protocols provided should be effective for the majority of patients. However, some broad guidelines in treating the following categories of pathology prevail.

Protocols – Frequency, Duty Cycle, Energy Density, Duration, etc.

Degenerative
Chronic
Traumatic
Neurogenic
Inflammatory
Autoimmune

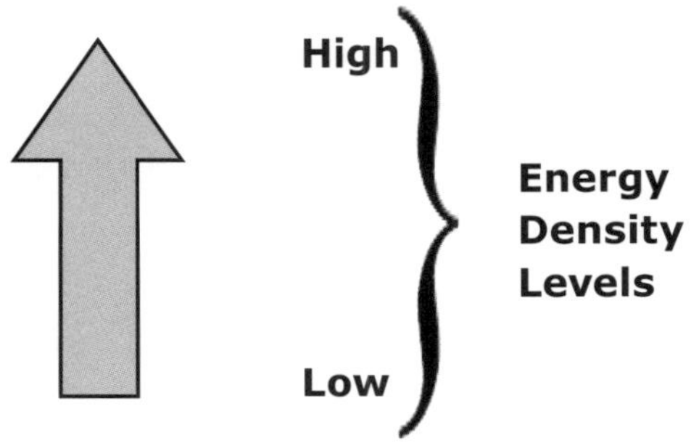

Application of Treatment Arrays

Although there is generally a focal point (accupoint) of pathology/pain, inevitably the area of involvement is much wider and deeper than generally surmised. We, therefore, always recommend that a wider tissue area be irradiated around the major focal point.

1. **Local:** Apply probe to the primary area of pathology.
2. **Nerve Root** of relevant dermatome as it exits the spinal cord.
3. **Peripheral Pain:** When treating areas of peripheral pain it is generally preferred to treat the nerve roots as they exit from the spinal canal in addition to the area where the pain sensation is localized. If the initial treatment of the localized area is successful this may not be necessary. However, therapeutic effectiveness is frequently enhanced when the nerve root origin is also treated. This is particularly valid with radiculitis where sciatic nerve pain is the subjective symptom but the appropriate application is over the nerve roots as they exit the spinal canal. Frequently, in treating localized lesions (i.e. carpal tunnel syndrome), it may be appropriate and extremely helpful to treat the cervical nerve root in conjunction with the localized therapy.
4. **Sandwich Approach:** (i.e. when treating the foot or wrist irradiate dorsal and plantar/palmar aspect during the same session). In areas such as the wrist, ankle, knee and foot, the therapeutic array should generally surround the entire joint. With the bones of the foot, particularly the talo-navicular, cuneiform and metatarsal regions, the "sandwich approach" is usually most effective with a portion of the therapy being applied dorsally, and similarly on the plantar aspect.
5. **Trigger or Accupoint:** Apply probe as directed over limited area
6. **Good Contact** between treatment arrays and tissue should always be maintained. This may require the gentle application of pressure keeping in mind that ventilation for proper cooling must continue. When strapping arrays into place, be sensitive with regard to the tissues at all times. Good contact without excessive pressure is important. Bindings should be snug but not too tight as this may occlude venous flow and lead to thrombosis.
7. **Tissues:** When treating any area, particularly a joint, attempt to irradiate all tissues involved. For example, the shoulder should be irradiated from the superior, anterior, posterior and lateral aspects with all arrays.
8. **Maintaining Cleanliness:** Always wash hands between treating patients. Utilize saran wrap or plastic casings when treating inguinal/axillary areas where higher bacterial counts exist. It is also advisable to cleanse the skin before the application of the arrays. Additionally, probes should be carefully cleaned with suitable antiseptic, between use on patients.
9. **Laser Operation:** When using the LD-I 75 and LD-I 200 treatment heads, the full effect of the therapy occurs after 1 minute of operation.
10. **Stage Three:** All areas can use the R-750 up to 1000/90 (frequency 1000Hz, duty cycle 90%) after other approaches have not produced a desirable result. Generally the IR-1500 is used in conjunction at 250/90 (frequency 250Hz, duty cycle 90%)

11. **Infrared 200 mW Laser Probe:** As evidence of Meditech's ongoing effort to improve the effectiveness of its therapy units along with the attendant protocols, we are pleased at this time to make available the 200mW Infrared Laser Probe. In the past year, Meditech in its clinical laboratory has carried out extensive testing utilizing the 200mW infrared probe. Whereas the 75mW infrared probe is satisfactory in most instances, the 200mW probe should be introduced in situations where the clinical status has reached a plateau, or more power is desirable. Instances where this is most applicable are cases with advanced osteoarthritis, particularly with stenosis of the spinal canal and foramen. Other conditions are degenerative osteoarthritis of the hips, knees, etc. and disc herniations. The 200mW probe can, of course, be run at any power level desired and time utilized can be reduced by 25-40% compared to the IR-75mW probe. Good clinical judgment as always, should prevail.

    The advantages of the 200mW probe are as follows:

    1) It can reduce the conventional treatment time by 25-40%
    2) It will be more effective in the therapy of more deeply located and chronic medical conditions.

12. **Red 25 mW Laser Probe:** Is applicable in the following conditions and usually in conjunction with the 75 mW IR probe:

    1. Tempero-Mandibular Joint Dysfunction
    2. Small joints of the hand
    3. Frontal and maxillary sinuses
    4. Trigeminal neuralgia
    5. Bell's Palsy

    This probe is frequently requested by acupuncturists.

13. **Treatment Heads:** The presciptions outlined in this book are prescribed with the LS-R 750, LS-I 1500, and LD-I 75 treatment heads. Each one of these treatment heads can be substituted with the following alternative treatment heads when appropriate (due to area covered and/or power density required):

Treatment Head	**Substitution Treatment Head**	**Comments**
LS-R 750	LS-R 250	Substitution treatment head covers 33% of the area. Same power density.
LS-R 750	SLD-R-500	Substitution treatment head covers approximately the same area but with 65% of the power density.
LS-R 750	SLD-R-1000 (under development)	Substitution treatment head covers more area but with 65% of the power density.
LS-I 1500	LS-I 500	Substitution treatment head covers 33% of the area. Same power density.
LS-I 1500	SLD-I-1000 (under development)	Substitution treatment head covers approximately the same area but with 65% of the power density.
LS-I 1500	SLD-I-2000	Substitution treatment head covers more area but with 65% of the power density.
LD-I 75	LD-I 200	Substitution treatment head covers same area and because of the higher power, reduces treatment time 25% - 40%.

Pulse Modulation

All the treatment arrays can be pulsed from one hertz per second to half a million hertz per second. Generally, we have confined our experience up to 10,000 hertz; however, we have initiated some studies to explore higher frequencies.

When the duty cycle is raised to 100% the pulse becomes continuous and you have what is known as a continuous wave (CW).

In our experience we usually operate the red arrays in continuous mode, at least initially, and pulse the infrared array. This may change with patient response or if a plateau is reached. Again, changes are based on clinical experience and judgement. For example, the patient may respond well at a frequency of 20 Hz and a duty cycle of 40%, but if the latter is increased to 60% and this results in pain, it should be reduced.

Always remember that all heads can be operated in pulsed or continuous mode.

Use of Arrays in Combination

Our standard procedure at this time is to use the red array in continuous mode followed by the infrared array pulsed and the infrared probe again in continuous mode. This appears to be satisfactory in most instances. On occasion, if treatment time is a factor, one can simply use the infrared array with or without the probe and for superficial lesions, the large surface red array with or without the probe. Again, these decisions are based on clinical experience and judgement (i.e. the human factor).

To summarize, in conditions such as dermal or superficial lesions, one array (red array) may be utilized effectively but with pathologies located further away from the dermal surface, e.g. arthritis of the spine, the infrared large surface array may be used by itself, with or without the infrared laser probe.

The permutations and combinations are infinite and the system was designed with these aspects in mind (i.e. unrestricted flexibility).

No matter how sophisticated the computer software program may be, a great deal of clinical judgement must always be exercised. For example, in the case of autoimmune disease and elderly patients, low frequencies and duty cycles are generally applicable initially. As the treatment progresses, larger doses may be required and are tolerated quite easily. Our standard treatment for most conditions is between 25 and 45 minutes, however, for back problems and pathological conditions of greater scope and depth, up to one hour or more may be utilized.

As in all medical practice, there are no absolutes and what we have provided are broad and reliable guidelines. Some knowledge pertaining to anatomy, physiology, physics and clinical medicine is important in maximizing the applicability of the BioFlex device. At all times one must be aware that individual tissue response varies and this factor cannot always be anticipated.

The manual presents reliable basic treatment protocols that should be successful in the majority of the patient population, relieving symptoms in over 75% of these patients. Customization will be required for the remainder, leading to overall improvement in excess of 90% and eventually 100%.

With the BioFlex System, an experienced therapist can rapidly learn to individualize (i.e. customize) protocols for each patient. Alternatively, the manual can be utilized for its basic directives.

The Concept of Clinical Laser Practice

- Laser Therapy is not designed to manage pain but to cure the cause.
- One should never operate for pain; prior to performing surgical procedures particularly if a clear cut diagnosis is not available, it is preferable to institute a course of laser therapy. Surgery can always be carried out at a later date, if necessary.
- Once a diagnosis has been established, and the protocols and expected outcomes have been explained to the patient, therapy should begin.
- No patient can improve unless therapy is initiated.
- Investigative procedures can be ordered at leisure and this should not preclude initiating treatment on the basis of a working diagnosis.
- When treatment plateaus are reached, as is sometimes the case, positive encouragement should be given. Adjusting protocols is generally appropriate at this point in order for healing to continue.
- Each day's aspect of the therapy should be explained to the patient in detail if required and the patient should be encouraged to continue treatment until positive results are achieved.
- Several conditions can be treated on the same visit simultaneously, if a sufficient number of therapeutic devices are available.
- Explain the need for continuing therapy or the consideration of a periodic maintenance program as indicated.
- Preferably, patients should be treated by the same therapist on each visit; building relationships engenders trust and contributes to the patient's comfort level.
- In the administration of laser therapy one should always present a positive ambience, a standard that should be prevalent in all medical practice.
- Laser Therapy does not conform to the regulatory criteria i.e. HMO's, governments, codes, etc. - from a clinical perspective neither do patients.
- These are just some of the important factors that we have found to be helpful in order to obtain positive clinical outcomes. Moreover, this approach constitutes a smoothly functioning seamless therapeutic environment.

In the literature and frequently in conversations one hears discussions regarding the "placebo effect" or the anecdotal aspect of therapy. Skeptics will always be skeptics. Despite them, it has been proven conclusively that Low Intensity Laser Therapy is the most exciting technology in the rehabilitation industry today. The healing power of Low Intensity Laser Therapy based on the interaction between light and cells offers a technology that is widely applicable and has unlimited healing power; it will enable clinicians to safely treat a wide variety of cellular pathologies without significant risk.

The 10 Commandments of Patient Care

Today society demonstrates a high degree of disregard for the individual. This is particularly regrettable in dealing with patients who are ill and as a result may demonstrate unacceptable behavior patterns. Whereas this is not their right, it is excusable on the basis of their pain and other symptoms and should therefore be disregarded. Aside from this there are certain principles that should be adhered to in patient management.

1. A human voice should answer the telephone at all times during clinic hours. Patients should not be kept waiting unduly on the telephone or at reception.

2. The response of the receptionist should be warm, friendly and courteous. Never react negatively to a patient no matter what the provocation may be. If you do so, you cease to be of any value to the healing process.

3. The temperature of the facility should be comfortable, the atmosphere bright and clean, magazines should be up to date and refreshments should be available.

4. Any reasonable request on the part of the patient should be carefully attended and engender a positive response. Attempt to satisfy patient requests even if they do not conform to the expected standard.

5. Eliminate the use of the words "no" and "sorry" as much as possible from your vocabulary. Even try "yes" once in a while; it works wonders.

6. Discussions should focus on the patient's problem, the therapeutic process and what may be expected. Carefully enumerate the ideal number of treatments, their frequency and anticipated result, at the same time explaining that there is variation between individuals.

7. Perform assessments in a friendly and relaxed fashion. Make sure that the patient is comfortable at all times.

8. Advise the patient of diagnosis, treatment plan and potential outcome in a realistic, positive manner. Whereas one should focus on the positive aspects of the situation do not avoid discussing potential negative factors. This approach also generates trust and confidence.

9. Background classical music is comforting and relaxing to most patients, not to mention staff. Sessions should consist of a soothing experience which will diminish the patient's apprehension and stress and is conducive to achieving the primary objective i.e. to heal the patient.

10. Always attempt to make the therapeutic experience seamless, including scheduling future visits to accommodate the patient.

This novel approach once prevalent will make everyone feel better; both office staff and more importantly the patient. As a consequence, patients will be more tolerant and compliant. Staff members will feel more of a participant and obtain a greater sense of personal gratification. It is easier to smile, be friendly and positive; it can also be part of the healing process.

Parameters

Frequency (Hz)
Duty Cycle (%) (Width of the pulse)
Power Density (mW)
Energy Density (J/cm^2)
Duration (sec)
Waveform
Helpful Hints

Parameters

Frequency (Hz)

When the system is used in "Modulation" "Mode of operation", frequency describes how many times (cycles) per second the waveform repeats. For example, the figure below shows a square wave repeating 2 times in one second.

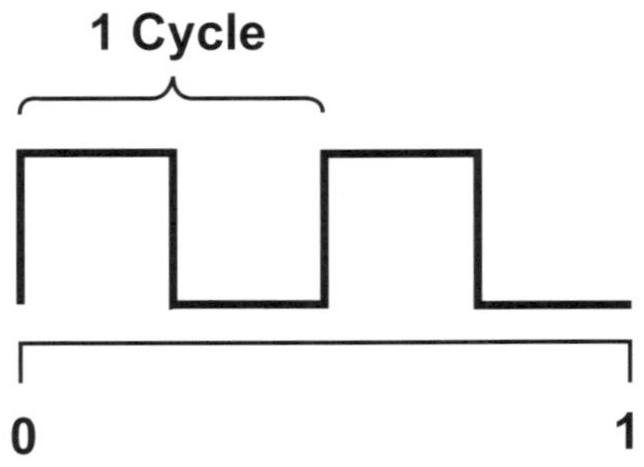

Therefore, the frequency of the above waveform is 2 cycles per second (c/s) or 2 Hertz (Hz).

Duty Cycle (%) (Width of the pulse)

When the system is used in "Modulation" "Mode of operation", duty cycle describes the percentage of time the waveform is functioning.

The figure below shows a square waveform with a duty cycle of 50% because it is on for half of its full time (1/2 x 100% = 50%).

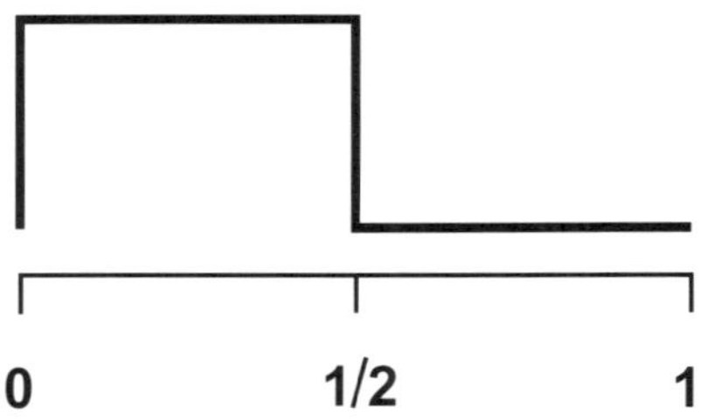

The figure below shows a square waveform with a duty cycle of 25% because it is on for 1/4 of its full time (1/4 x 100% = 25%).

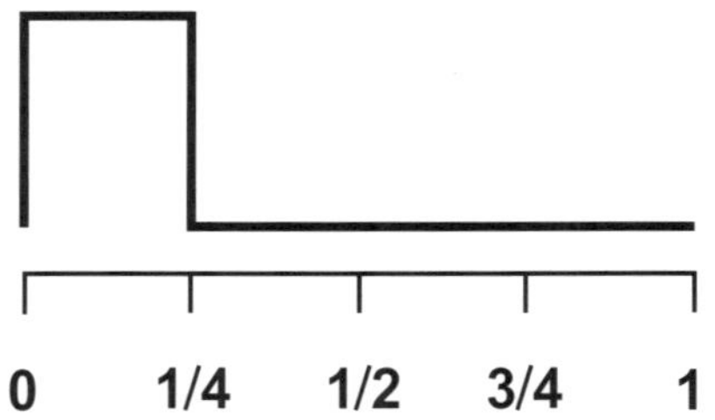

Power Density (mW)

Measured in milliWatts per square centimeter (mW/cm^2), power density describes the amount of light delivered over the treatment area. For example, if a 60 Watt (equals 60,000mW) light delivers all its light to a $10cm^2$ area, the power density is:

$60{,}000 \div 10 = 6{,}000 mW/cm^2$

Energy Density (J/cm2)

Indicates the amount of power divided by the area (see power density), multiplied by time (or duration). This is measured in Joules per square centimeter (J/cm^2). For example, if a 60 Watt (W) light delivers all its light to a $10cm^2$ area for 10 seconds, the power density is:

$$60 \div 10 \times 10 = 60 J/cm^2$$

Duration (sec)

The length of time of the treatment.

Waveform

When the system is used in "Modulation" "Mode of operation", there are three waveforms that can be selected: square, sine and triangle. The waveform controls the output intensity of the laser or SLD. For example, a square wave controls the intensity by either turning on and off the laser or SLD, without intermediate states. A sine or triangle wave controls the intensity by turning on and off the laser or SLD slowly

Pictorially, the waveforms are shown below:

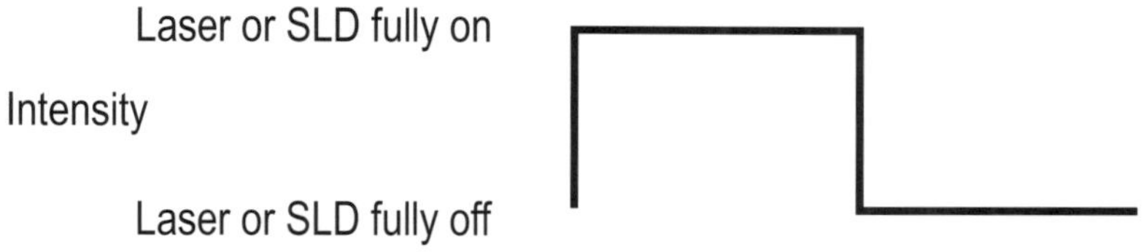

Square Wave

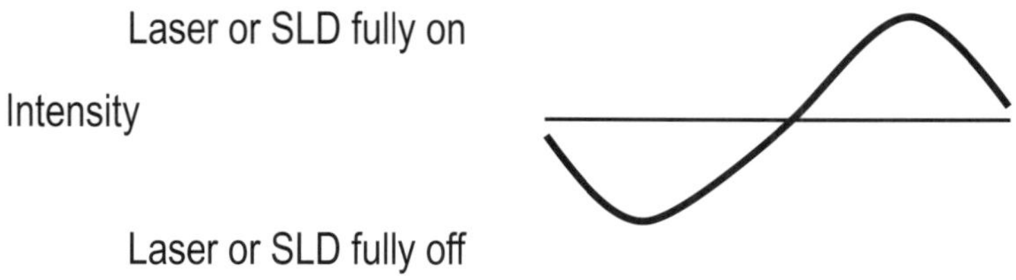

Sine Wave

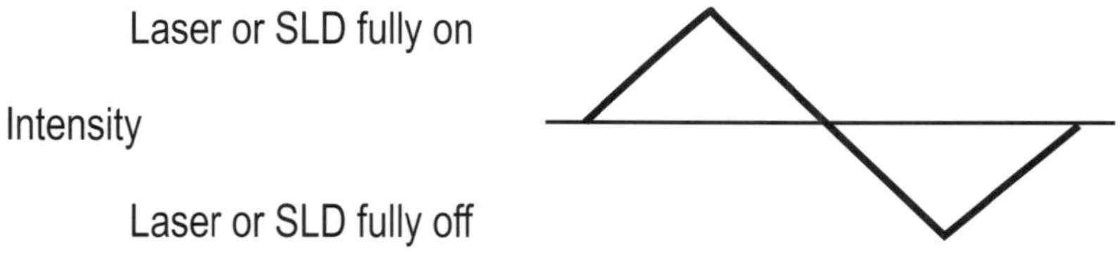

Triangle Wave

Helpful Hints!

1) The 200mW laser probe may be substituted in most situations at Stage II or Stage III.

2) All arrays may be run in pulsed or continuous mode.

3) Massage / Heat Packs may be applied in all cases.

4) Length of treatment is always subject to individual variation.

5) No protocol is absolute and the system is totally flexible allowing an infinite number of permutations and combinations with regard to treatment parameters.

6) Creativity and good clinical judgement are the keynotes at all times.

Prescriptions

Cervical Spine
Thoracic Spine
Lumbosacral
Shoulder Joint
Rotator Cuff Injury
Elbow Joint
Epicondylitis
Wrist
Hand/Digits
Hip Joint
Adductor Muscle Injuries (Muscle Origin Tear)
Thigh and Leg Muscle Injuries
Knee Joint
Lower Extremity
Ankle and Foot
Achilles Tendonitis
Plantar Fascitis
Headaches
Facial Pain
Tempero-Mandibular Joint Dysfunction
Herpes Zoster
Rheumatoid Arthritis
Lymphaedema
Fibromyalgia
Dermatological Applications
Generic I Degenerative Osteoarthritis
Generic II Tendonitis
Generic III Inflammatory Conditions
Generic IV Autoimmune Conditions

Cervical Spine

- Soft Tissue Injuries
- Degenerative Osteoarthritis
- Cervical Radiculopathy
- Facet Joint Syndrome
- Disc Herniation with or without Radiculopathy

Stage One:

Treatment Head	*Frequency*	*Duty Cycle*	*Duration (minutes)*
LS-R 750	CW		6/6
LS-I 1500	10-20	20-70	7/7
LD-I 75	CW		6-10

Stage Two:

Treatment Head	*Frequency*	*Duty Cycle*	*Duration (minutes)*
LS-R 750	100	90	6/6
LS-I 1500	50	50-90	7/7
LD-I 75	CW		6-10

Stage Three:

Treatment Head	*Frequency*	*Duty Cycle*	*Duration (minutes)*
LS-R 750	250-1000	90	6/6
LS-I 1500	50-250	80-90	7/7
LD-I 75	CW or 100	90	6-10

Treatment Tips:

1) Treat from occiput to T2 vertically and transversely from C4-T3.
2) Place probe to areas of pathology (accupoints); generally over the para-cervical muscles from C1-T3 as clinically indicated.
3) May also treat vertically and then with two oblique positions.
4) In advanced cases we have found that aditional therapy to the lateral aspects of the C-spine utilizing the R-250 and IR-500 arrays enhances effectiveness.
5) One can generally add 6 minutes of each or more on the lateral aspect (C2-6) using protocols similar to those prescribed. This will increase total treatment time by 24 minutes but is useful in advanced cases of degenerative osteoarthritis.
6) The 200mW laser probe may be substituted on the basis of clinical response at the Stage Two or Stage Three level.

Cervical Spine

A

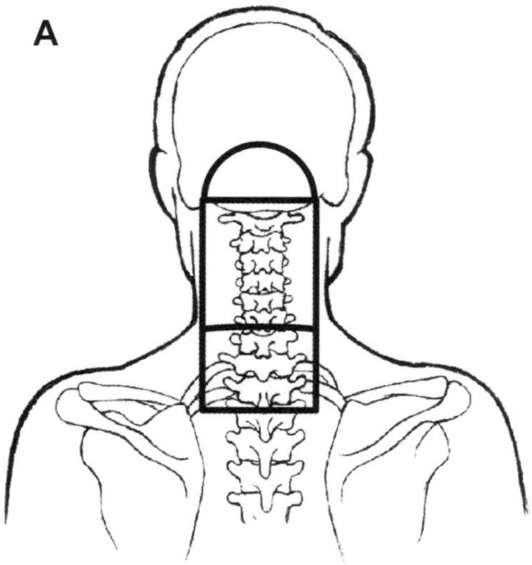

B

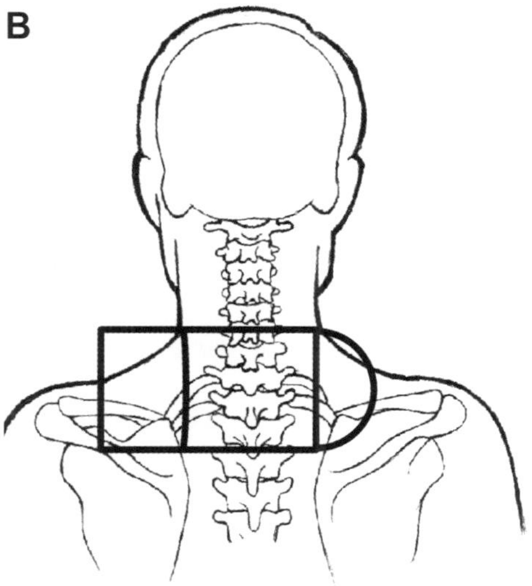

C

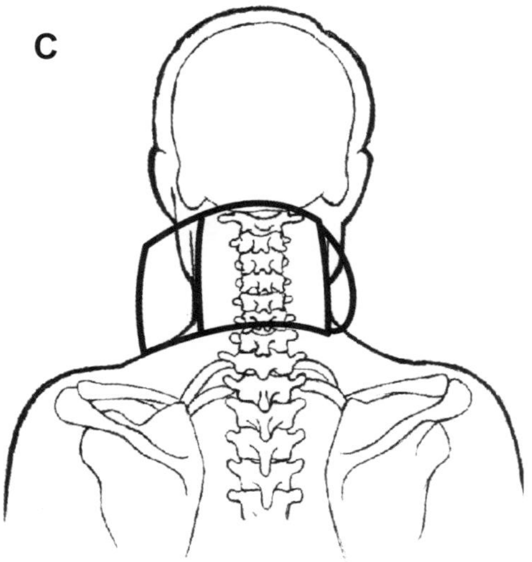

D

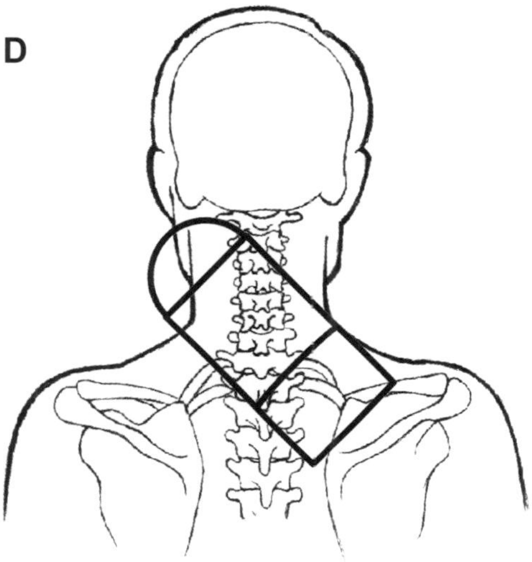

E

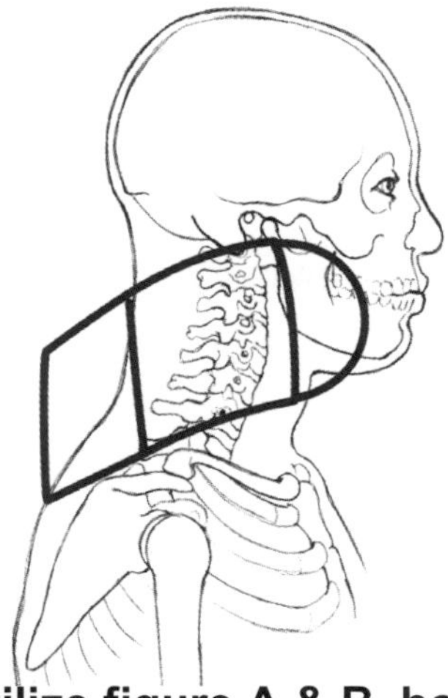

F

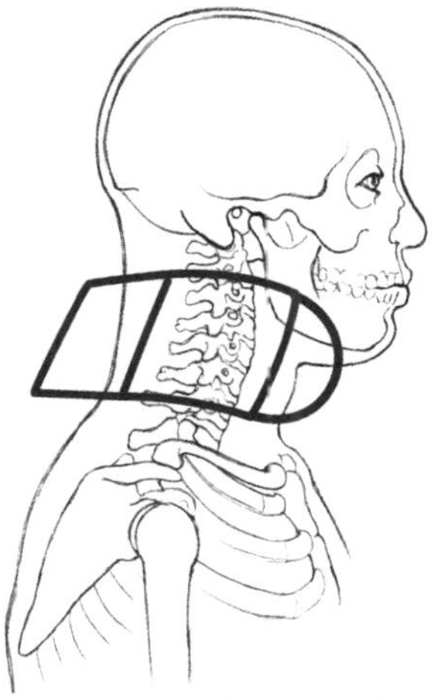

Normally utilize figure A & B, however, anatomically, figure C may be preferable to A. Also consider D, E and F.

D. May use 750mW & 1500mW arrays obliquely or 250mW & 500mW arrays; the latter two preferably applied to the lateral aspect of the C-Spine transversely (the 750mW & 1500mW arrays may be too large.)

Thoracic Spine

- Kyphosis
- Myofascitis
- Compression Fractures
- Degenerative Osteoarthritis

Stage One:

Treatment Head	*Frequency*	*Duty Cycle*	*Duration (minutes)*
LS-R 750	CW	50-90	6/6
LS-I 1500	50		7/7
LD-I 75	CW		6-10

Stage Two:

Treatment Head	*Frequency*	*Duty Cycle*	*Duration (minutes)*
LS-R 750	CW	80-90	6/6
LS-I 1500	50		7/7
LD-I 75	CW		6-10

Stage Three:

Treatment Head	*Frequency*	*Duty Cycle*	*Duration (minutes)*
LS-R 750	250-1000	80-90	6/6
LS-I 1500	250-5000	80-90	7/7
LD-I 75	CW or 100	90	6-10

Treatment Tips:

1) Depending on the extent of pathology, treat 30-60 minutes.
2) In most situations after initial 2-3 treatment sessions 200mW IR laser probe may replace 75mW IR laser probe.
3) In myofascitis may start (Stage One) with LS-R 750 continuous wave and LS-I 1500 at 50 Hz frequency and 60% duty cycle.

Thoracic Spine

A

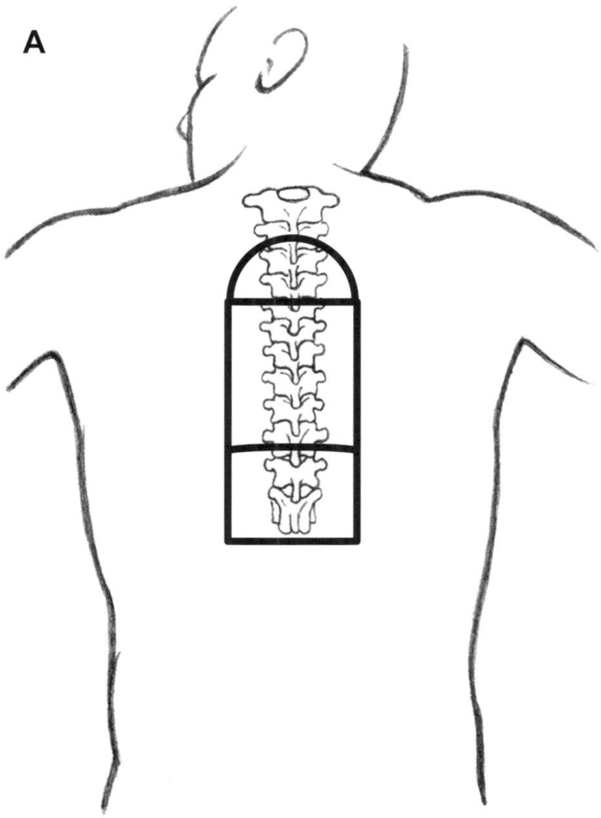

B

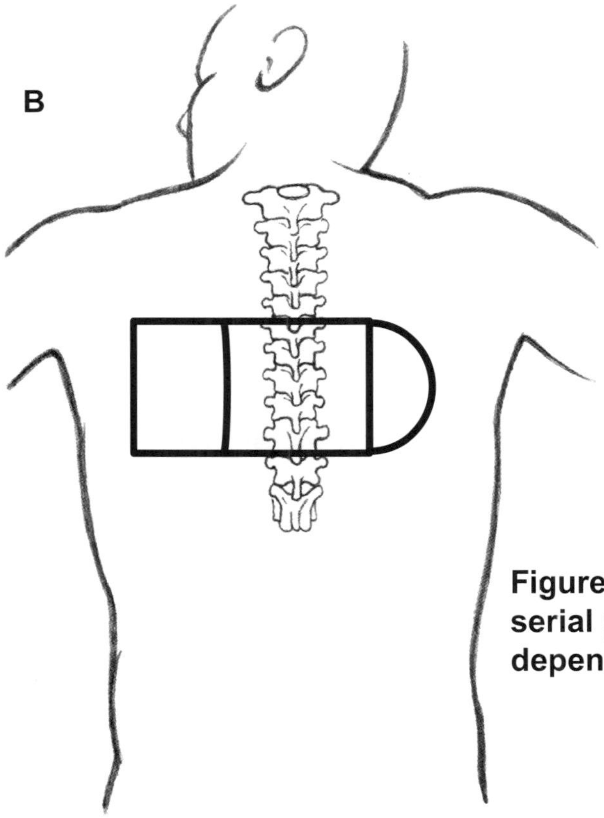

1

2 — Position

3

Figure B may be used in serial positions 1,2 & 3 depending on the pathology.

Lumbosacral

- Degenerative Osteoarthritis with Spinal/Foraminal Stenosis
- Disc Herniation with Radiculopathy
- Facet Joint Syndrome
- Sacroiliac Joint Dysfunction
- Soft Tissue Injuries

Stage One:

Treatment Head	*Frequency*	*Duty Cycle*	*Duration (minutes)*
LS-R 750	CW		8/8/8 or 10/10
LS-I 1500	50	50-90	10/10/10
LD-I 75	CW		6-10

Stage Two:

Treatment Head	*Frequency*	*Duty Cycle*	*Duration (minutes)*
LS-R 750	CW		8/8/8 or 10/10
LS-I 1500	250	90	10/10/10
LD-I 75	CW		6-10

Stage Three:

Treatment Head	*Frequency*	*Duty Cycle*	*Duration (minutes)*
LS-R 750	250-1000	80-90	8/8/8 or 10/10/10
LS-I 1500	500-10,000	80-90	10/10/10
LD-I 75	CW or 100	90	6-10

Treatment Tips:

1) Unless symptoms are localized, one hour of treatment is advisable.
2) Use probe over facet joints, disc or nerve root as indicated clinically.
3) With both Red and Infrared Large Surface Array, use 10/10 minutes as in position A unless radiation of pain to lower extremities is present. Then place array vertically for 8 minutes & obliquely to both left & right side as illustrated in B.
4) May use LS-I 1500 vertically over L-S spine for 6-10 min in position C.

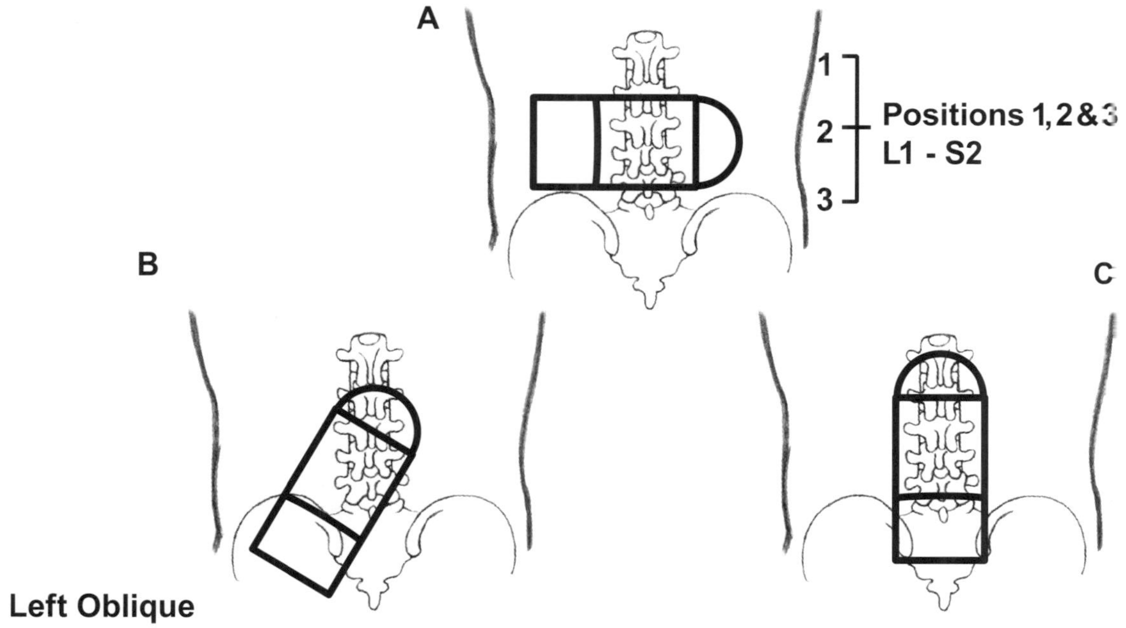

Figures A, B & C

Lumbar spine: May use both right and left oblique positions, if radiation of symptoms extends to both lower extremities.

Probes are applied over focal points following the application of Large Surface Array.

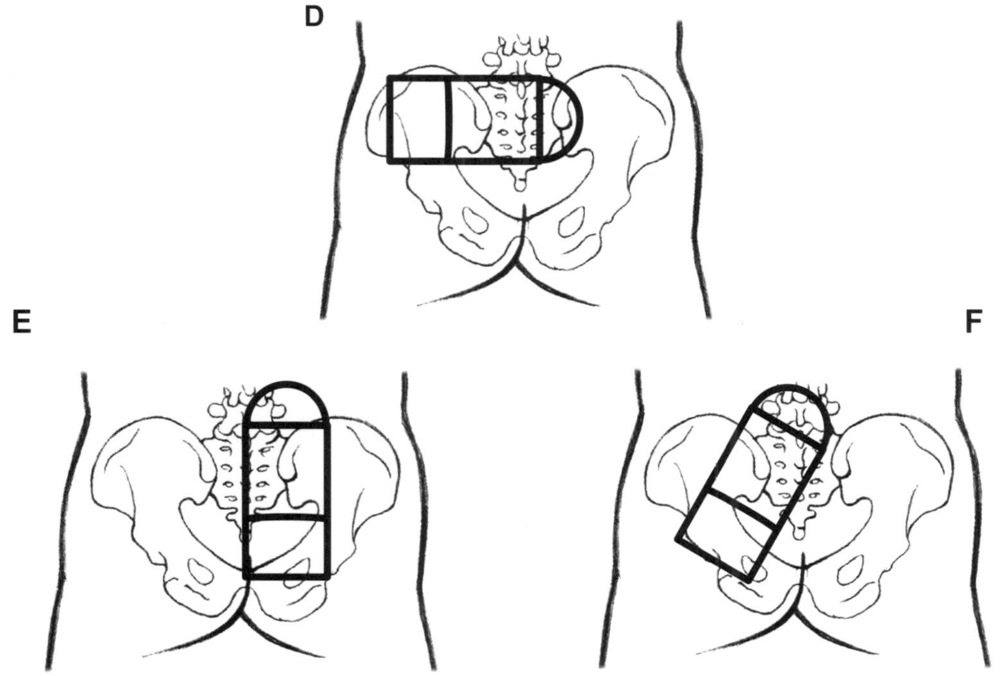

Figures D, E & F

S.I. Joint: Apply as appropriate using a combination of any two positions followed by Infrared Probe over the S.I. Joint.

Shoulder Joint

- Acromioclavicular Joint Dysfunction; (Trauma, Separation, Arthritis)
- Ligamentous injury
- Impingement Syndrome
- Adhesive Capsulitis (Frozen Shoulder)
- Tendonitis/Bursitis
- Repetitive Stress Injury
- Tendinosis

Stage One:

Treatment Head	*Frequency*	*Duty Cycle*	*Duration (minutes)*
LS-R 750	CW		6/6
LS-I 1500	10-50	30-80	6/6/6
LD-I 75	CW		6-8

Stage Two:

Treatment Head	*Frequency*	*Duty Cycle*	*Duration (minutes)*
LS-R 750	100	90	6/6
LS-I 1500	50	50-90	6/6/6
LD-I 75	CW		6-8

Stage Three:

Treatment Head	*Frequency*	*Duty Cycle*	*Duration (minutes)*
LS-R 750	250-1000	90	6/6
LS-I 1500	250	80-90	6/6/6
LD-I 75	CW or 100	70-90	6-10

Treatment Tips:

1) Stage one may start at 10 Hz and 20-50 % duty cycle with LS-I 1500.

Shoulder Joint

A

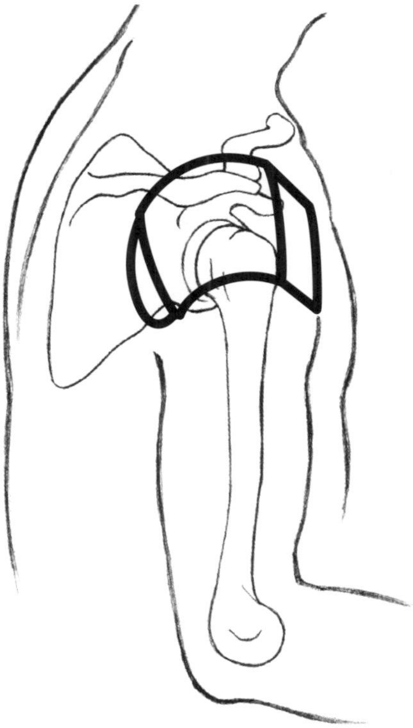

B

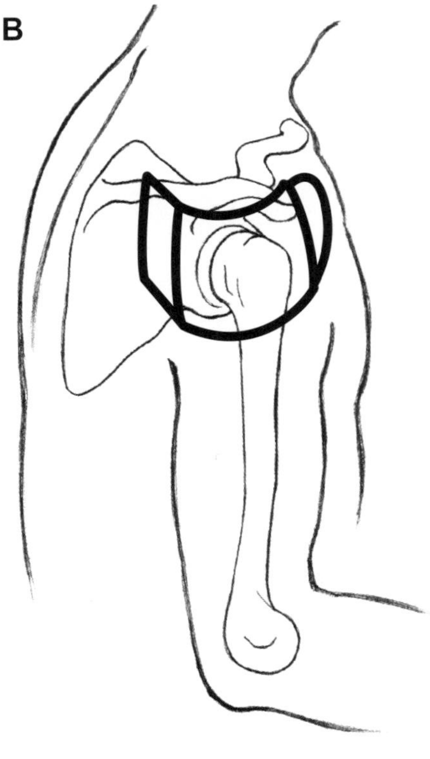

C

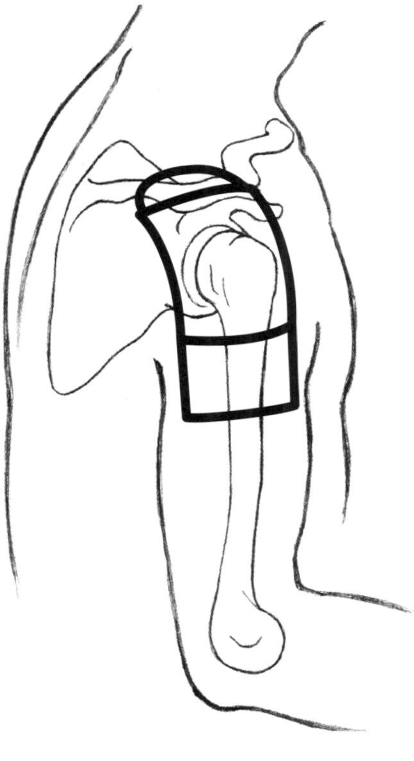

Usually apply Large Surface Red Array as in figures A & B and Infrared Array as in figures A, B & C. Follow with Infrared Probe over focal points (ports accessible to joint). i.e., anterior & posterior joint capsule, subacromial area and deltoid.

Rotator Cuff Injury

Stage One:

Treatment Head	*Frequency*	*Duty Cycle*	*Duration (minutes)*
LS-R 750 LS-I 1500 LD-I 75	CW 10-20 CW	40-80	6/6 6/6/6 6

Stage Two:

Treatment Head	*Frequency*	*Duty Cycle*	*Duration (minutes)*
LS-R 750 LS-I 1500 LD-I 75	CW 50 CW	80	6/6 6/6/6 6

Stage Three:

Treatment Head	*Frequency*	*Duty Cycle*	*Duration (minutes)*
LS-R 750	1000	90	6/6
LS-I 1500	250	80	6/6/6
LD-I 75	CW or 100	70-90	6

Treatment Tips:

1) As an adjunct; weekly massage therapy is recommended with this and most other conditions.
2) With all shoulder and upper extremity problems examine and X-ray C-spine to determine concomitant pathologies which may also require treatment.

Rotator Cuff Injury

A

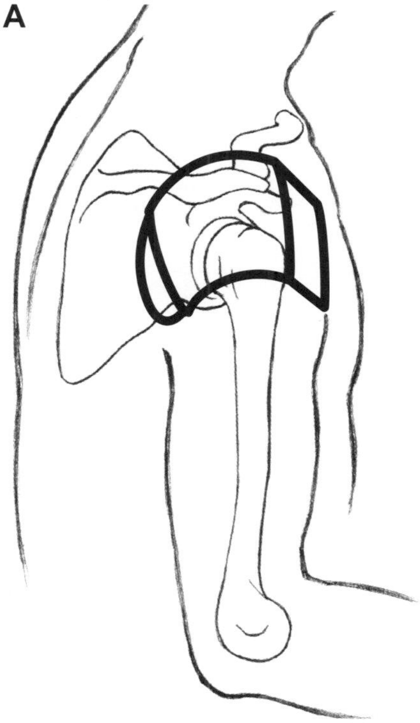

B

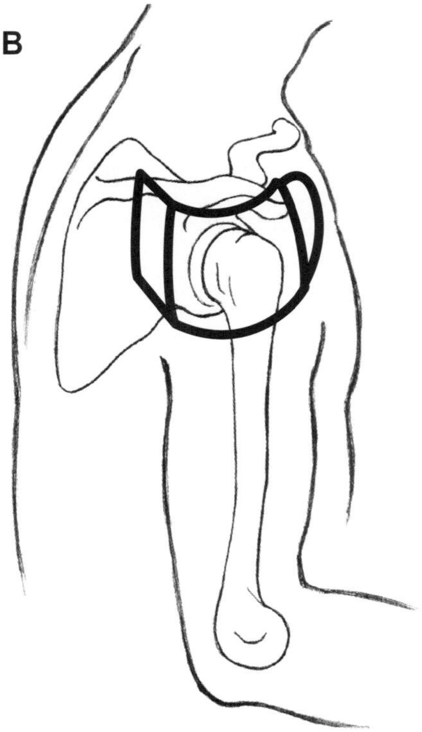

C

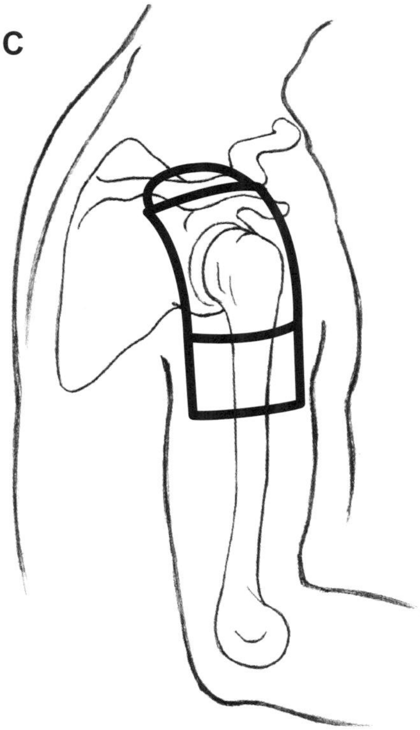

Apply Large Surface Red Array as in figures A & B and Infrared Array as in figures A, B & C. Follow with Infrared Probe over focal points (ports accessible to joint).
i.e., anterior & posterior joint capsule, subacromial area, and deltoid.

Elbow Joint

- Biceps/Triceps Tendonitis
- Olecranon Bursitis
- Degenerative Osteoarthritis
- Ulnar Nerve Pathologies

Stage One:

Treatment Head	*Frequency*	*Duty Cycle*	*Duration (minutes)*
LS-R 750	CW		6/6
LS-I 1500	10-20	40-80	6/6
LD-I 75	CW		6

Stage Two:

Treatment Head	*Frequency*	*Duty Cycle*	*Duration (minutes)*
LS-R 750	CW		6/6
LS-I 1500	20-70	30-90	6/6
LD-I 75	CW		6

Stage Three:

Treatment Head	*Frequency*	*Duty Cycle*	*Duration (minutes)*
LS-R 750	500-1000	70-90	6/6
LS-I 1500	50-100	80-90	6/6
LD-I 75	CW or 100	90	6-10

Elbow Joint

A

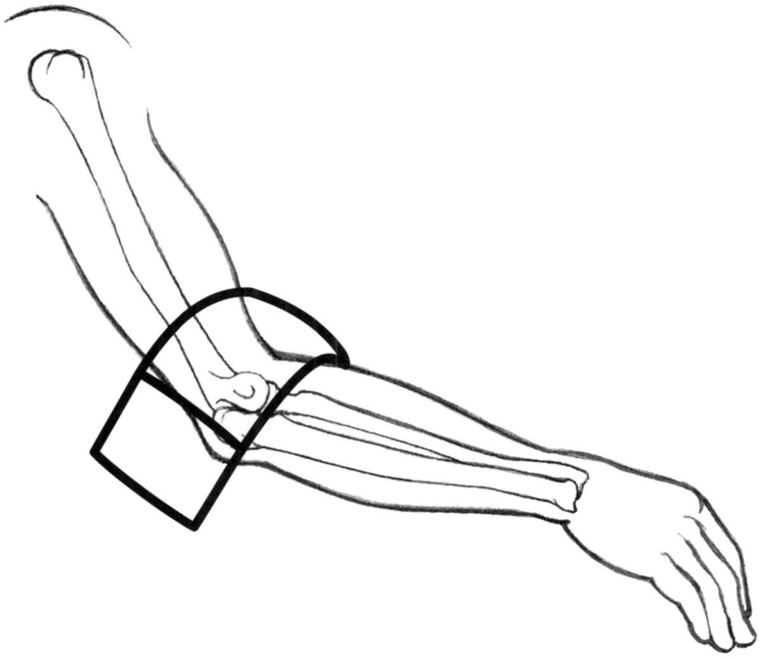

B

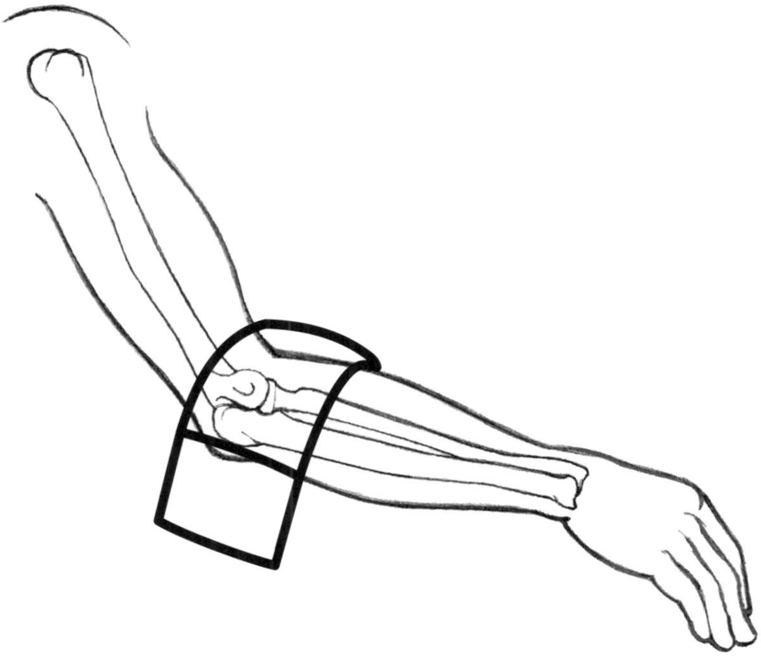

Apply Large Surface Red Array as in figure A if radiation of symptoms is to the arm; or as in figure B if radiation of the symptoms is to the forearm. Otherwise utilize a position that is central over the joint.
Treat around the entire circumference of the joint based on clinical findings.

Epicondylitis

Stage One:

Treatment Head	*Frequency*	*Duty Cycle*	*Duration (minutes)*
LS-R 750 LS-I 1500 LD-I 75	CW 10-20 CW	40-80	8 14 6

Stage Two:

Treatment Head	*Frequency*	*Duty Cycle*	*Duration (minutes)*
LS-R 750 LS-I 1500 LD-I 75	CW 50 CW	50-90	8 14 6

Stage Three:

Treatment Head	*Frequency*	*Duty Cycle*	*Duration (minutes)*
LS-R 750	100-1000	90	8
LS-I 1500	250	80	14
LD-I 75	CW or 100	70-90	6

Treatment Tips:

1) Move arrays proximally if triceps or brachio-radialis is involved and distally if the flexor/extensor muscles are involved. In either case, cover the medial and/or lateral epicondyle.
2) Applicable for both medial and lateral epicondylitis.

Epicondylitis

A

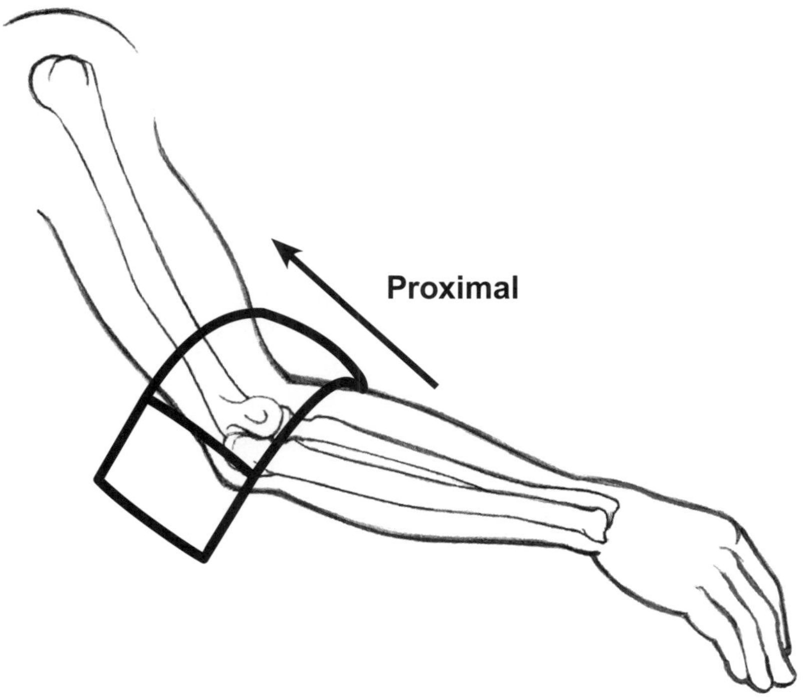

B

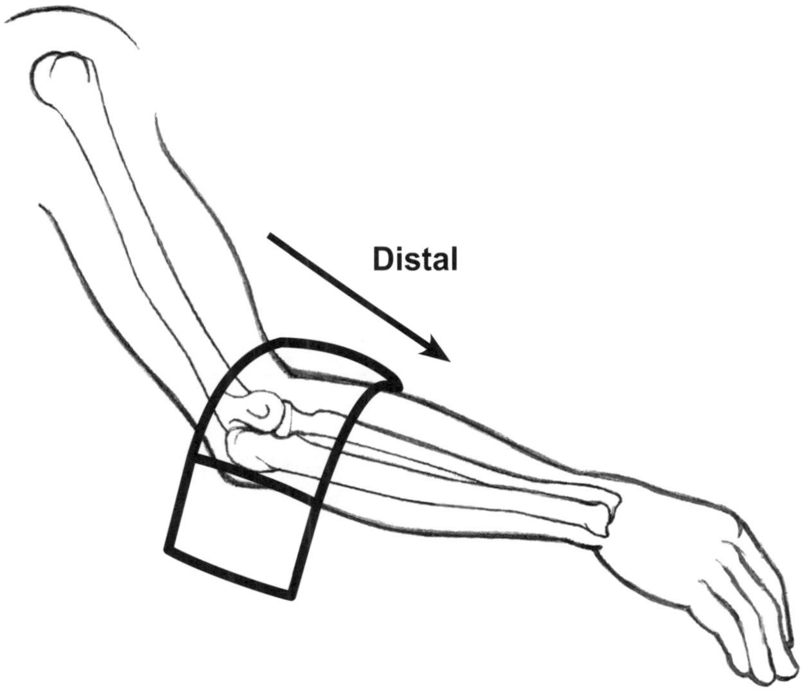

Wrist

- Carpal Tunnel Syndrome
- Peripheral Nerve Compression
- Fractures
- Degenerative Osteoarthritis

Stage One:

Treatment Head	*Frequency*	*Duty Cycle*	*Duration (minutes)*
LS-R 750	CW		10
LS-I 1500	10-20	40-70	14
LD-I 75	CW		6

Stage Two:

Treatment Head	*Frequency*	*Duty Cycle*	*Duration (minutes)*
LS-R 750	100	90	10
LS-I 1500	50	50-90	14
LD-I 75	CW		6

Stage Three:

Treatment Head	*Frequency*	*Duty Cycle*	*Duration (minutes)*
LS-R 750	250-1000	90	10
LS-I 1500	250-500	70-90	14
LD-I 75	CW or 100	90	6-10

Treatment Tips:

1) Apply probe from area proximal to flexor retinaculum to mid palm following the course of the median nerve for Carpal Tunnel Syndrome.
2) In all situations LD-I 200 may be substituted if clinically indicated.

Wrist

A

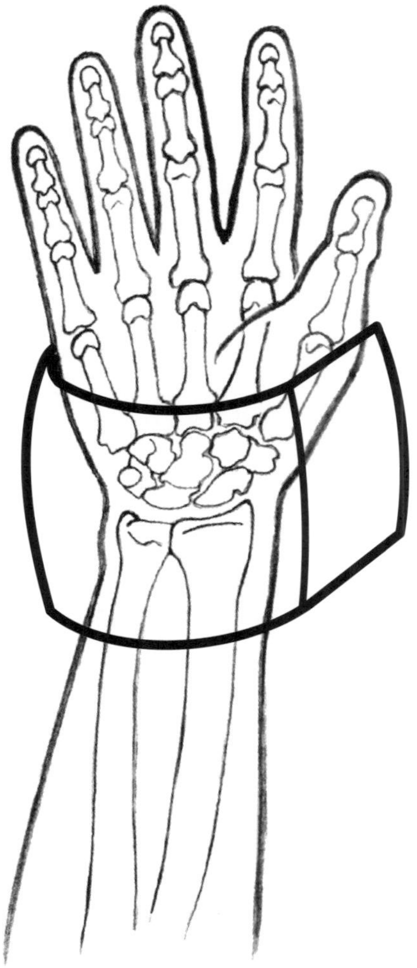

B

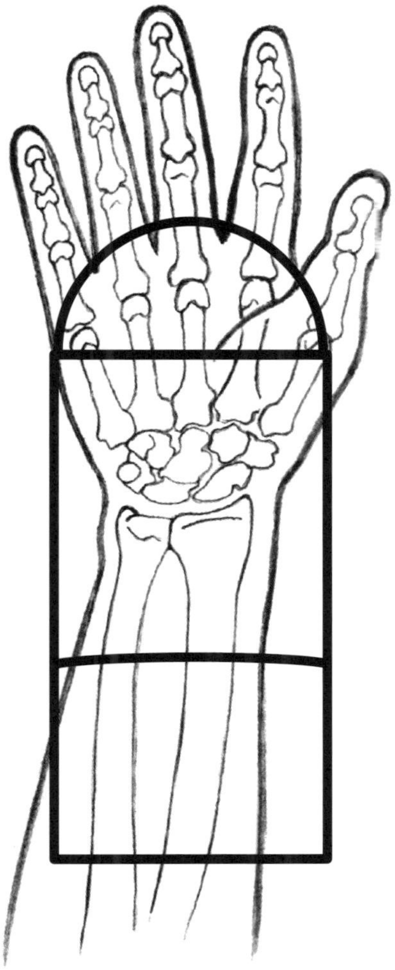

Can use Large Surface Array as in figure A, over dorsal and palmar aspect, deleting B as indicated.

May also use portion of treatment time (30-40%) as in illustration B. On occasion may apply over dorsal aspect.

Hand/Digits

- Dupuytran's Contracture
- Soft Tissue Injuries
- Degenerative Osteoarthritis
- De Quervains Disease
- Metacarpal Fractures

Stage One:

Treatment Head	*Frequency*	*Duty Cycle*	*Duration (minutes)*
LS-R 750	CW		10
LS-I 1500	50	70	14
LD-I 75	CW		6-10

Stage Two:

Treatment Head	*Frequency*	*Duty Cycle*	*Duration (minutes)*
LS-R 750	100	90	10
LS-I 1500	50	90	14
LD-I 75	CW		6-10

Stage Three:

Treatment Head	*Frequency*	*Duty Cycle*	*Duration (minutes)*
LS-R 750	250-1,000	70-90	10
LS-I 1500	250-5,000	70-90	14
LD-I 75	CW or 100	90	6-10

Treatment Tips:

1) When treating digits always use laser probe around entire circumference of joints.
2) Apply for longer duration over surface most involved (palmar vs. dorsal aspect).

Hand/Digits

A

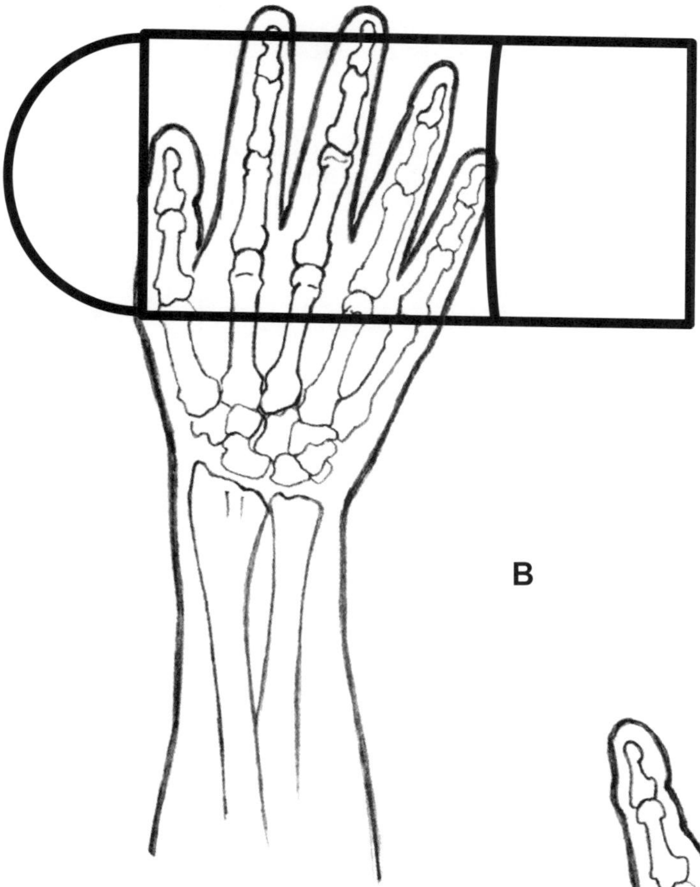

B

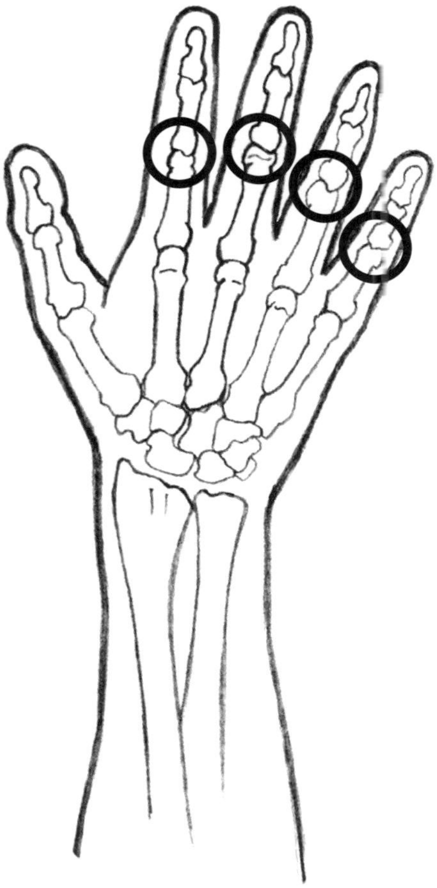

Fingers, Thumb & Palm

A: Red and/or Infrared Array

B: Application of probe to MP and IP joints.

Hip Joint

- Trauma/Ligamentous/Fracture
- Capsulitis/Synovitis
- Degenerative Osteoarthritis

Stage One:

Treatment Head	*Frequency*	*Duty Cycle*	*Duration (minutes)*
LS-R 750 LS-I 1500 LD-I 75	CW 50 CW	60-90	8/8/8 10/10/10 3/3/3

Stage Two:

Treatment Head	*Frequency*	*Duty Cycle*	*Duration (minutes)*
LS-R 750 LS-I 1500 LD-I 75	500 250 CW	90 90	8/8/8 10/10/10 3/3/3 or more

Stage Three:

Treatment Head	*Frequency*	*Duty Cycle*	*Duration (minutes)*
LS-R 750 LS-I 1500 LD-I 75	250-1000 5000 CW or 100	90 80-90 90	8/8/8 10/10/10 3/3/3 or more

Treatment Tips:

1) One should utilize three laser treatments per week, one hour of massage weekly and daily non-weight bearing /stretching exercises as tolerated.
2) The IR 75 laser probe is applied for nine minutes (three minutes each) over the anterior, lateral and posterior ports of the hip joint.
3) Aquatherapy & massage / stretching here as in all conditions, accelerates the healing process.
4) With hip pathologies in most cases back problems co-exist and also require investigation and treatment.

Hip Joint

A

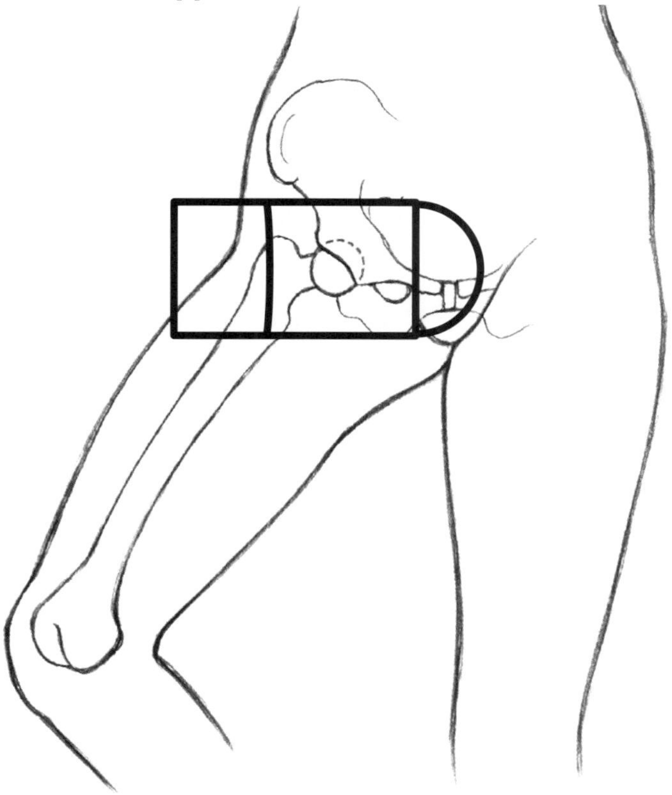

B

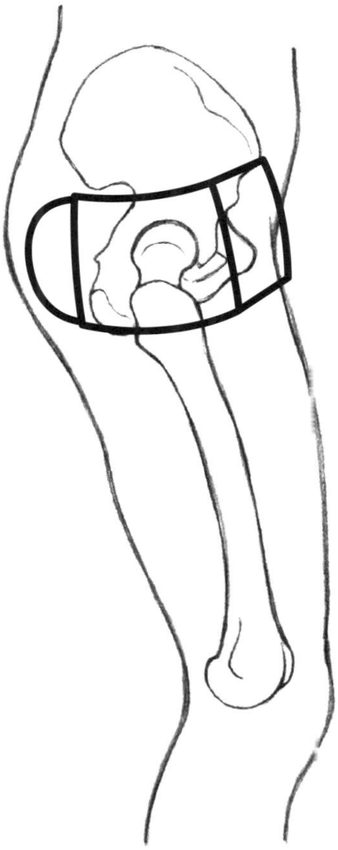

C

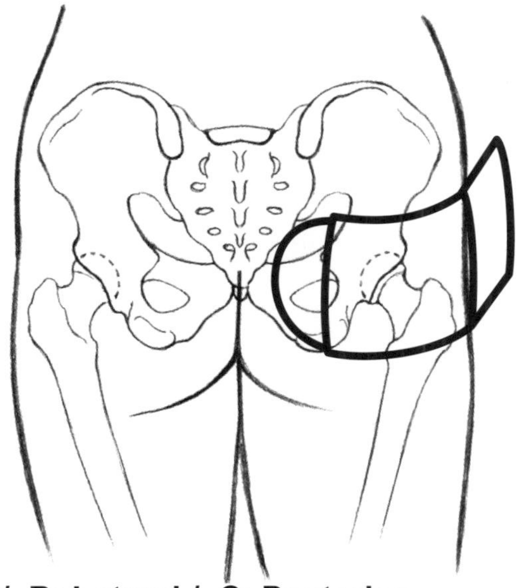

A: Anterior / B: Lateral / C: Posterior

Three points of approach to the hip joint.

As in all instances, use Large Surface Red Array followed by Infared Array and finally Infrared Probe.

Adductor Muscle Injuries (Muscle Origin Tear)

- Adductor Longus/Brevis/Magnus

This may also involve inguinal ligament pathologies, osteitis pubis and injury to rectus abdominis muscle insertion; similar for ilio-psoas, piriformis and ilio-tibial band problems.

Stage One:

Treatment Head	*Frequency*	*Duty Cycle*	*Duration (minutes)*
LS-R 750 LS-I 1500 LD-I 75	CW 50 CW	70	10 14 6-10

Stage Two:

Treatment Head	*Frequency*	*Duty Cycle*	*Duration (minutes)*
LS-R 750	100-250	90	10
LS-I 1500	50	90	15
LD-I 75	CW		6-10

Stage Three:

Treatment Head	*Frequency*	*Duty Cycle*	*Duration (minutes)*
LS-R 750	250-1000	90	10
LS-I 1500	250	90	15
LD-I 75	CW or 100	90	6-10

Treatment Tips:

1) Usually 30 minutes is sufficient but prolonged treatment time may be used to get results more quickly. <u>Irradiate widely!</u>

Adductor Muscle

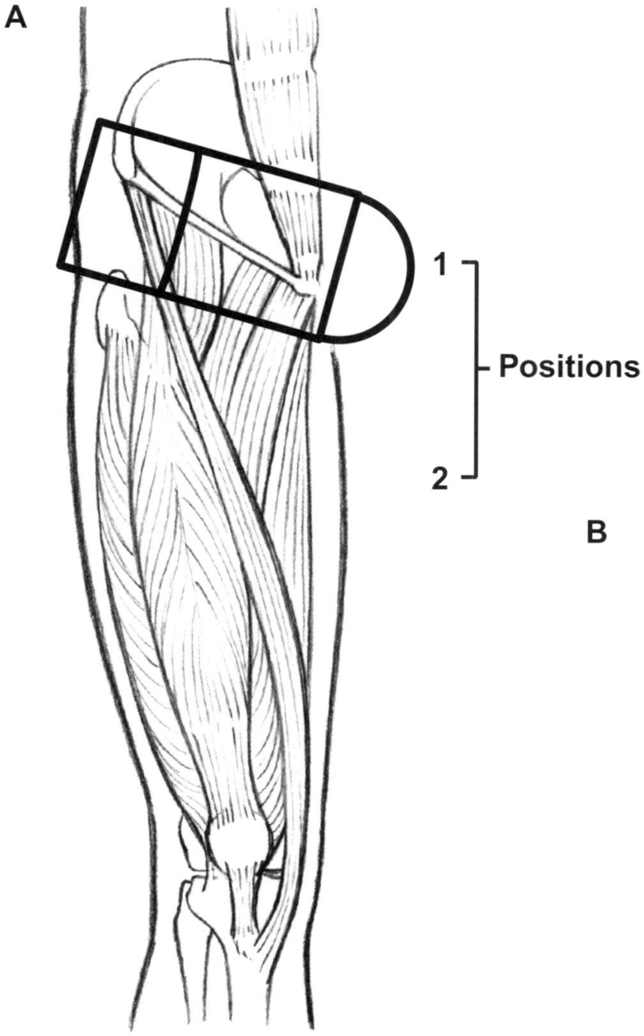

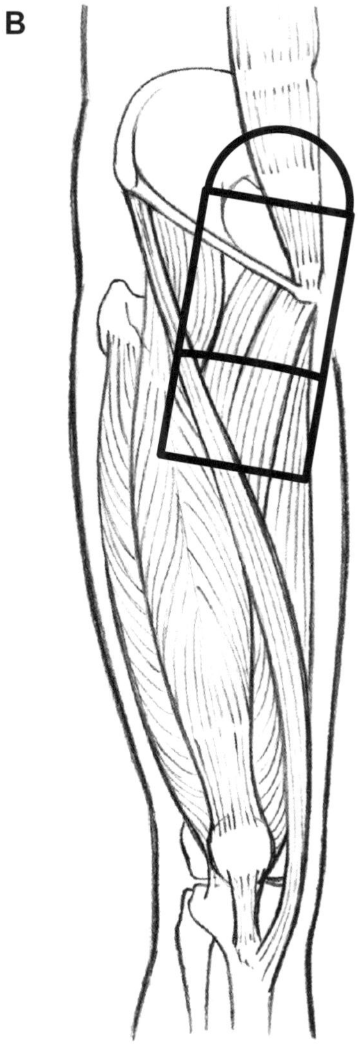

May apply Large Surface Array as in figure A or B in serial positions.

Apply A distally & B laterally for stage 2.

Thigh and Leg Muscle Injuries

- Hamstrings; Biceps Femoris, Semitendinosus, Semimembranosus
- Quadriceps; Rectus Femoris, Vastus Medialis, Vastus Intermedius, Vastus Lateralis, Psoas Major, Iliacus
- Sartorius

Stage One:

Treatment Head	*Frequency*	*Duty Cycle*	*Duration (minutes)*
LS-R 750	CW	60-90	10
LS-I 1500	50		15
LD-I 75	CW		6-10

Stage Two:

Treatment Head	*Frequency*	*Duty Cycle*	*Duration (minutes)*
LS-R 750	250	90	10
LS-I 1500	50	90	15
LD-I 75	CW		6-10

Stage Three:

Treatment Head	*Frequency*	*Duty Cycle*	*Duration (minutes)*
LS-R 750	1000	90	10
LS-I 1500	250	80-90	15
LD-I 75	CW or 100	90	6-10

Treatment Tips:

1) N.B. Thrombophlebitis must always be ruled out.
2) Depending on the extent of pathology, one hour of treatment may be required.
3) Laser appicable but patient should be on anticoagulants if possibility of embolic phenomena exists.

Thigh and Leg Muscles

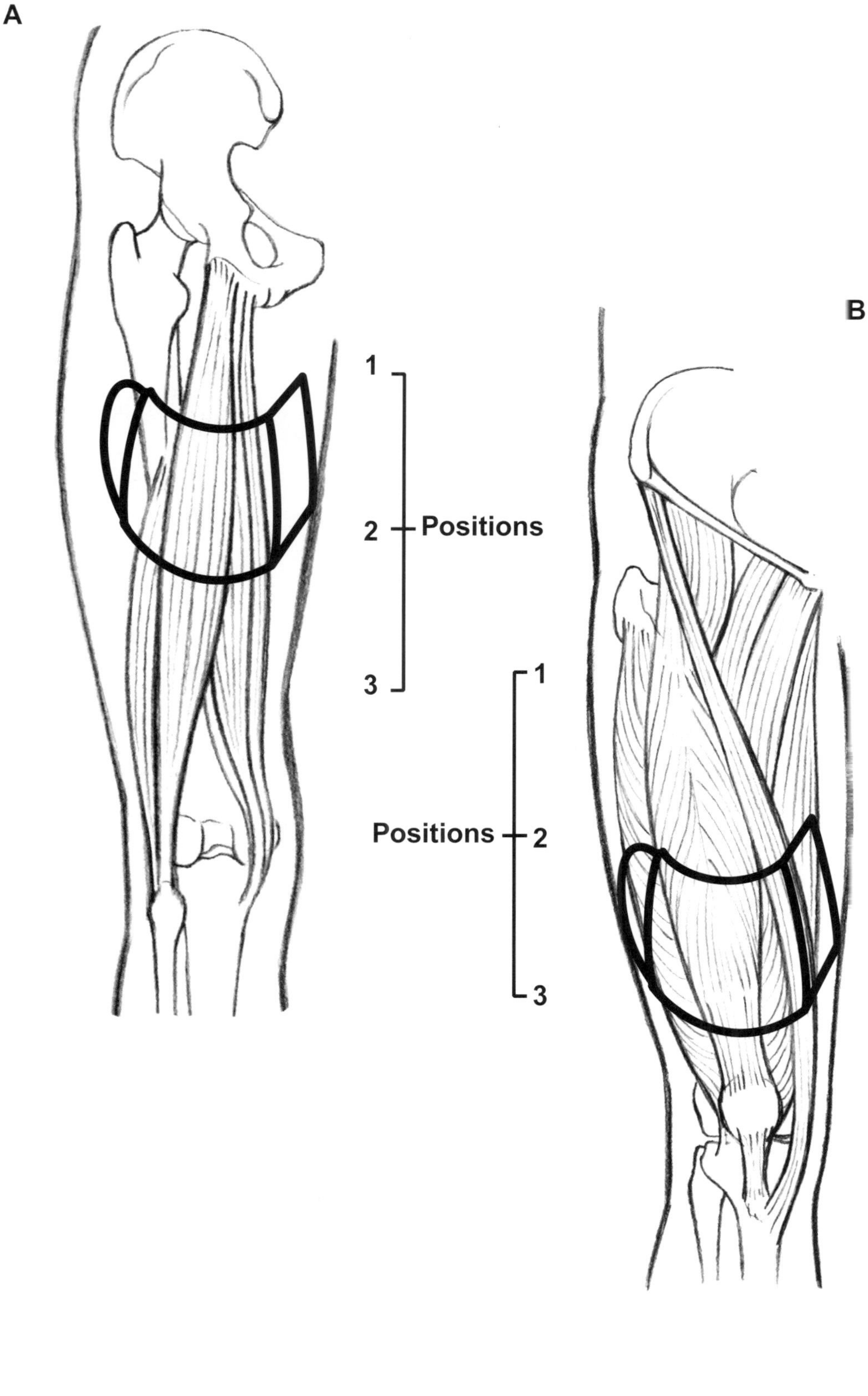

A: Hamstrings; Position 1, 2 & 3

B: Quadriceps mechanism injuries; similar placements may be utilized.

Knee Joint

- Ligamentous Injuries
- Meniscal Tears
- Supra/Infrapatellar Tendonitis
- Tendinosis
- Degenerative Osteoarthritis
- Chondromalacia Patella
- Osgoode-Schlatter Disease

Stage One:

Treatment Head	***Frequency***	***Duty Cycle***	***Duration (minutes)***
LS-R 750	CW		8
LS-I 1500	50	50-90	8/8
LD-I 75	CW		6-8

Stage Two:

Treatment Head	***Frequency***	***Duty Cycle***	***Duration (minutes)***
LS-R 750	100-250	90	8
LS-I 1500	250	70-90	8/8
LD-I 75	CW		6-8

Stage Three:

Treatment Head	***Frequency***	***Duty Cycle***	***Duration (minutes)***
LS-R 750	250-1000	80-90	8
LS-I 1500	250-5000	70-90	8/8
LD-I 75	CW or 100	90	6-10

Treatment Tips:

1) Generally thirty minutes is sufficient, however one hour may be required with large knees and extensive pathology. Treat four quadrants or, two anterior and one over the popliteal space as clinical assessment dictates, particularly in post knee-replacements with extensive induration and edema.
2) Treat around the entire circumference of the knee. 40-60% of the duration of the treatment is directed at the compartment most severely afflicted (usually the medial compartment). The remaining therapy is apportioned to the patellar and lateral components and the popiteal space as indicated. Both large red and infrared arrays are utilized as well as the laser probe. This maneuver provides better penetration into the knee joint and therefore is more effective
3) It should be noted that generally the knee is best treated in an extended position at 110–120°, (i.e. 20-30° beyond the knee at a right angle as seen in Figures B&C). For penetration to the posterior aspect of the patella and the patellar compartment, flexion of the knee to 90° or more may be advisable and treat circumferentially around patella.

Knee Joint

A

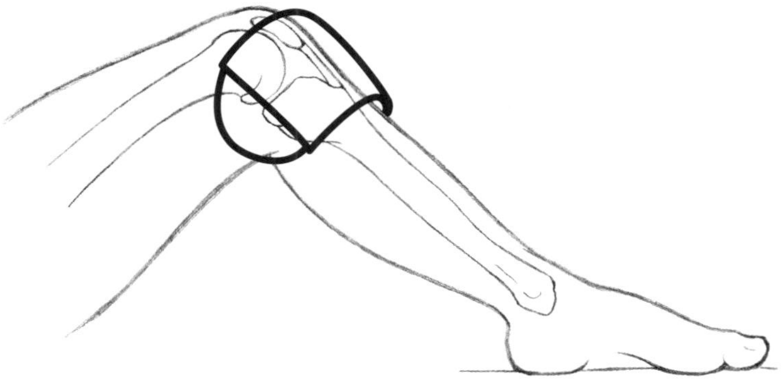

B

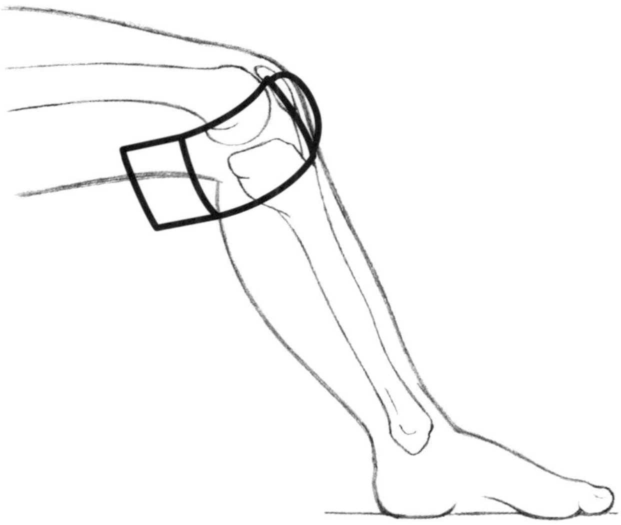

C

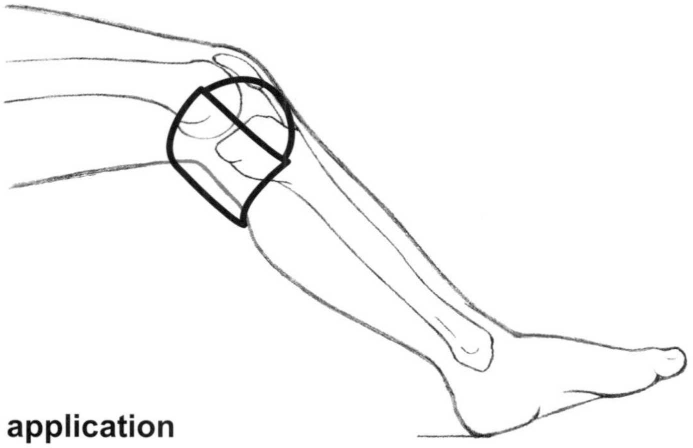

A: Central anterior application

B: Medial application

C: Central posterior application (popliteal space)

Large Surface Red Array are usually placed over medial/lateral compartments and popliteal space (circumferentially)

Emphasis of treatment using laser probe focused on the compartment most severely affected.

Above approach preferable however central position may be emphasized with osteomalacia patella, infrapatellar ligament problems and Osgood-Schlatter Disease. Generally though medial and lateral placements overlapping are preferable.

Lower Extremity

- Gastrocnemius (Medial and Lateral Heads)
- Soleus
- Anterior Tibial Compartment Syndrome
- Soft Tissue Injuries
- Myositis/Tendonitis
- Fractures

Stage One:

Treatment Head	***Frequency***	***Duty Cycle***	***Duration (minutes)***
LS-R 750 LS-I 1500 LD-I 75	CW 50 CW	60-90	6/6 6/6 6

Stage Two:

Treatment Head	***Frequency***	***Duty Cycle***	***Duration (minutes)***
LS-R 750 LS-I 1500 LD-I 75	100 50 CW	90 90	6/6 6/6 6

Stage Three:

Treatment Head	***Frequency***	***Duty Cycle***	***Duration (minutes)***
LS-R 750 LS-I 1500 LD-I 75	250-1000 250 CW or 100	90 80-90 90	6/6 6/6 6-10

Treatment Tips:

1) May require up to one hour if extensive area is involved.
2) Treat 30-60 minutes over the entire area with R 750 and IR 1500 treatment arrays with Anterior Tibial Compartment Syndrome and other soft tissue inflammatory processes.
3) If no acupoints exist then the laser probe may not be necessary.

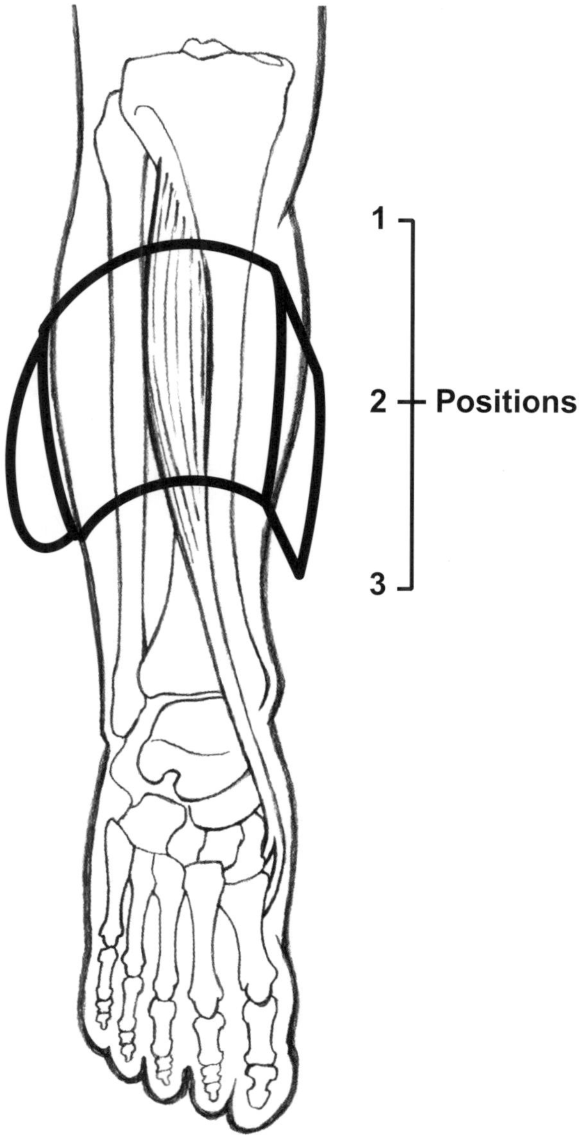

Position 1, 2 & 3 may be utilized in anterior tibial compartment syndrome and other problems as indicated.

Ankle and Foot

- Degenerative Osteoarthritis
- Neuropathy of the Foot
- Tarsal Tunnel Syndrome
- Morton's Neuroma
- Soft Tissue Injuries
- Stress Fracture
- Metatarsalgia
- Biomechanical Problems

Stage One:

Treatment Head	*Frequency*	*Duty Cycle*	*Duration (minutes)*
LS-R 750	CW		10
LS-I 1500	50	70	15
LD-I 75	CW		5

Stage Two:

Treatment Head	*Frequency*	*Duty Cycle*	*Duration (minutes)*
LS-R 750	100-250	90	6/6
LS-I 1500	50	90	6/6
LD-I 75	CW		6

Stage Three:

Treatment Head	*Frequency*	*Duty Cycle*	*Duration (minutes)*
LS-R 750	250-1000	90	6/6
LS-I 1500	250	80-90	6/6
LD-I 75	CW or 100	70-90	6

Treatment Tips:

1) Surround the joint with arrays where appropriate and possible from the anatomical perspective.
2) With Neuropathy may start at lower levels ie. LS-R 750 at 10 Hz and 50% duty cycle/ LS-I 1500 at 20 Hz and 30% duty cycle.

A

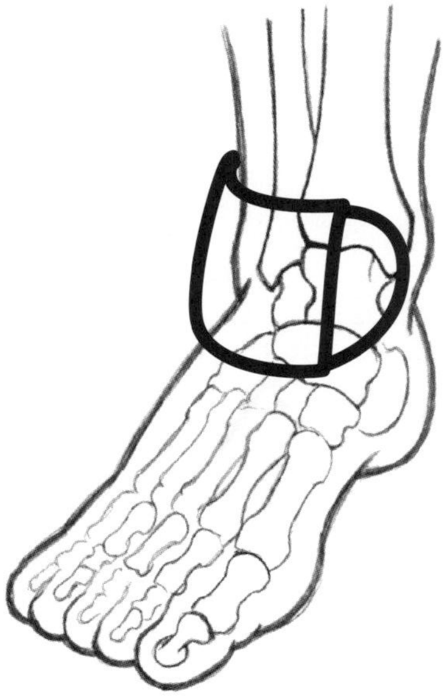

B

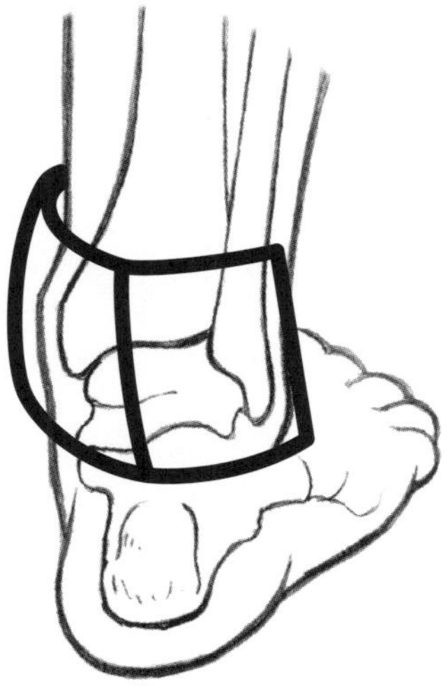

C

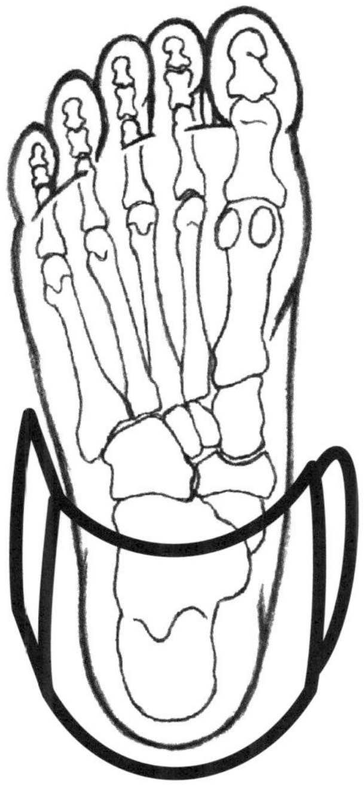

D

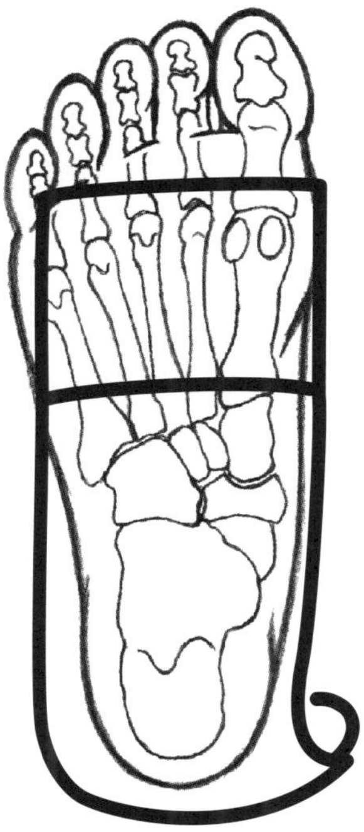

A is applicable for lateral and anterior approaches (i.e., ligamentous injuries, effusions, etc.)

B is appropriate for medial and posterior problems.

C and D are appropriate for a variety of problems as additional approaches (i.e. fascitis, calcaneal pathologies, degenerative osteoarthritis, etc.)

Achilles Tendonitis

Stage One:

Treatment Head	*Frequency*	*Duty Cycle*	*Duration (minutes)*
LS-R 750	10-50	50	6/6
LS-I 1500	10-20	30-80	7/7
LD-I 75	CW		6-8

Stage Two:

Treatment Head	*Frequency*	*Duty Cycle*	*Duration (minutes)*
LS-R 750	100	90	6/6
LS-I 1500	50	70-90	7/7
LD-I 75	CW		6-8

Stage Three:

Treatment Head	*Frequency*	*Duty Cycle*	*Duration (minutes)*
LS-R 750	250-1000	90	6/6
LS-I 1500	250	80-90	7/7
LD-I 75	CW or 100		6-8

Treatment Tips:

1) These protocols apply to all tendonitis problems.

Achilles Tendonitis

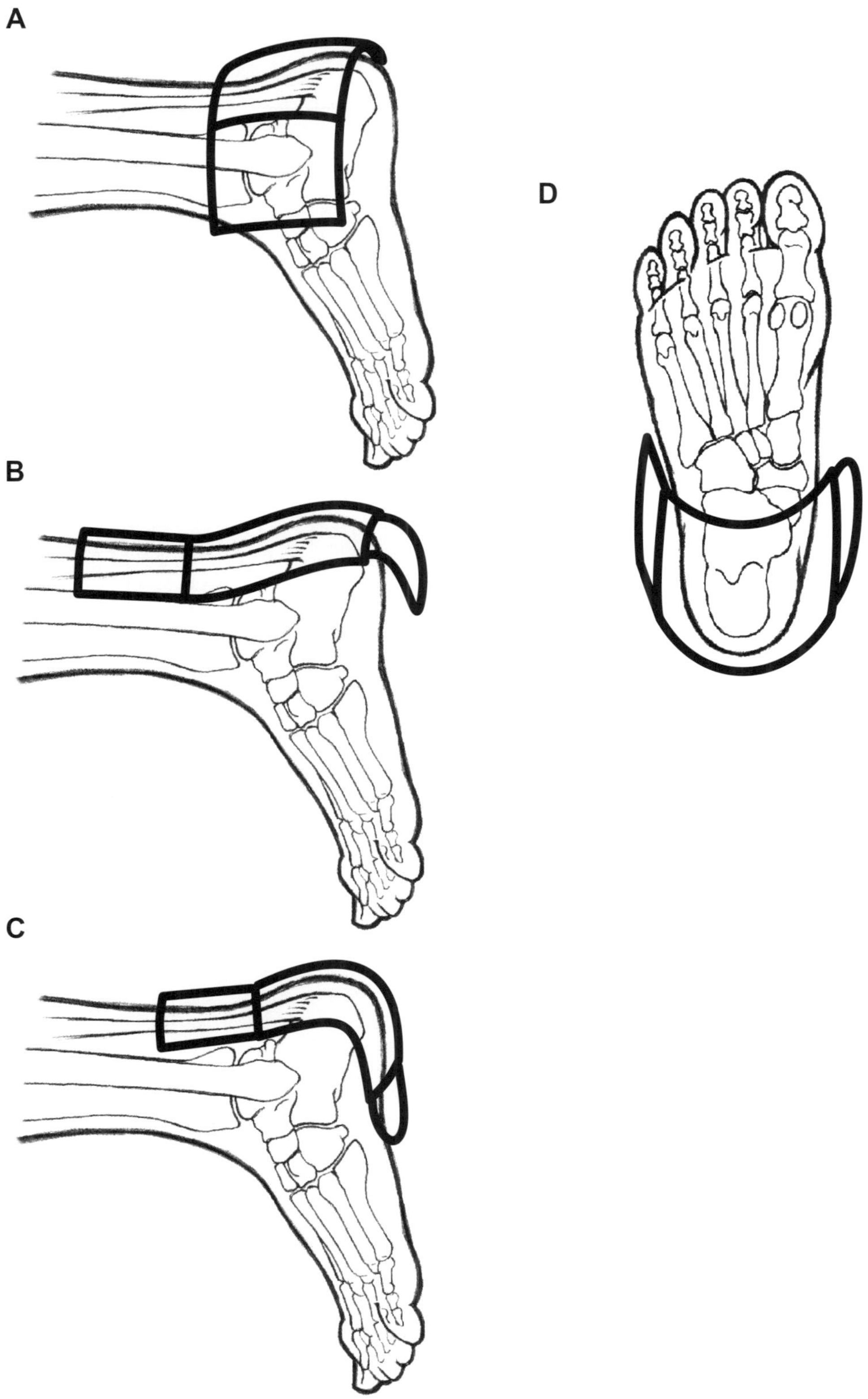

Plantar Fascitis and Achilles Tendonitis (AT) are frequently associated conditions.

In these instances, the position of the Large Surface Array can be applied to AT insertion and heel pad simultaneously, as in C. Otherwise, apply Arrays as indicated above.

Plantar Fascitis

Stage One:

Treatment Head	*Frequency*	*Duty Cycle*	*Duration (minutes)*
LS-R 750 LS-I 1500 LD-I 75	CW 10-20 CW	30-90	6/6 6/6 6

Stage Two:

Treatment Head	*Frequency*	*Duty Cycle*	*Duration (minutes)*
LS-R 750	100	80	6/6
LS-I 1500	50	70-90	6/6
LD-I 75	CW		6

Stage Three:

Treatment Head	*Frequency*	*Duty Cycle*	*Duration (minutes)*
LS-R 750	100-1000	90	6/6
LS-I 1500	250	80-90	6/6
LD-I 75	CW or 100	90	6

Treatment Tips:

1) Area of treatment may include insertion of the achilles tendon and/or peroneus brevis/longus tendons and/or plantar fascia.
2) Treat in accordance with the extent of the pathology.
3) May also involve the fascia of the arch and forefoot.

Plantar Fascitis

A

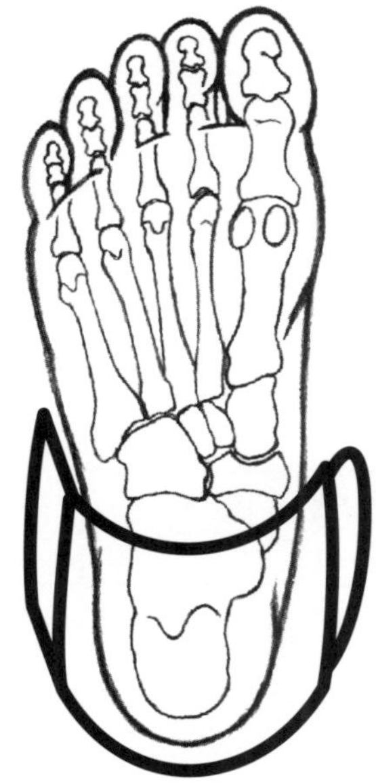

C

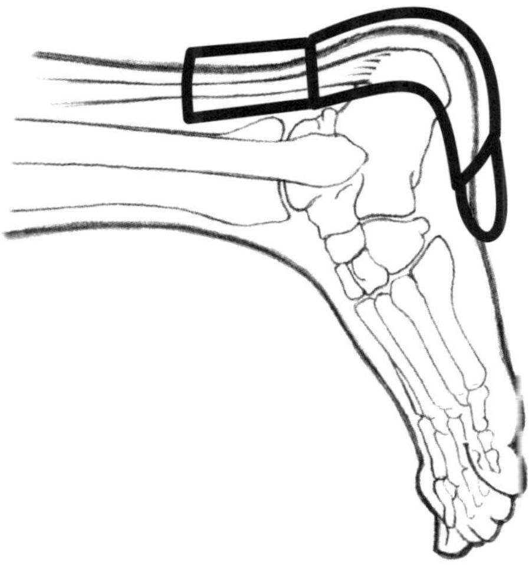

B

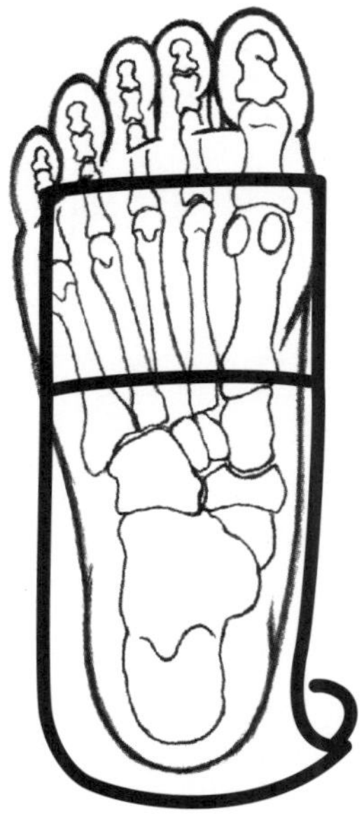

Follow the prescribed protocol, focusing on the painful areas extensively with the Infrared Probe.

Headaches

- Migraine
- Tension
- Cervicogenic
- Post Concussion
- Non-specific

Stage One:

Treatment Head	*Frequency*	*Duty Cycle*	*Duration (minutes)*
LS-R 750 LS-I 1500 LD-I 75	CW 5-20 CW	20-50	5/5 7/7 6

Stage Two:

Treatment Head	*Frequency*	*Duty Cycle*	*Duration (minutes)*
LS-R 750 LS-I 1500 LD-I 75	100 20-50 CW	90 60-80	5/5 7/7 6

Stage Three:

Treatment Head	*Frequency*	*Duty Cycle*	*Duration (minutes)*
LS-R 750 LS-I 1500 LD-I 75	100-500 250 CW or 100	90 80-90 70-80	5/5 7/7 6

Treatment Tips:

1) You may start with the IR at 5/20 Hz if the tissue status is felt to be questionable and increase gradually from there as indicated.
2) May also utilize 3 position approach vertical and oblique to right and left instead of transverse (Figure D).

Headaches

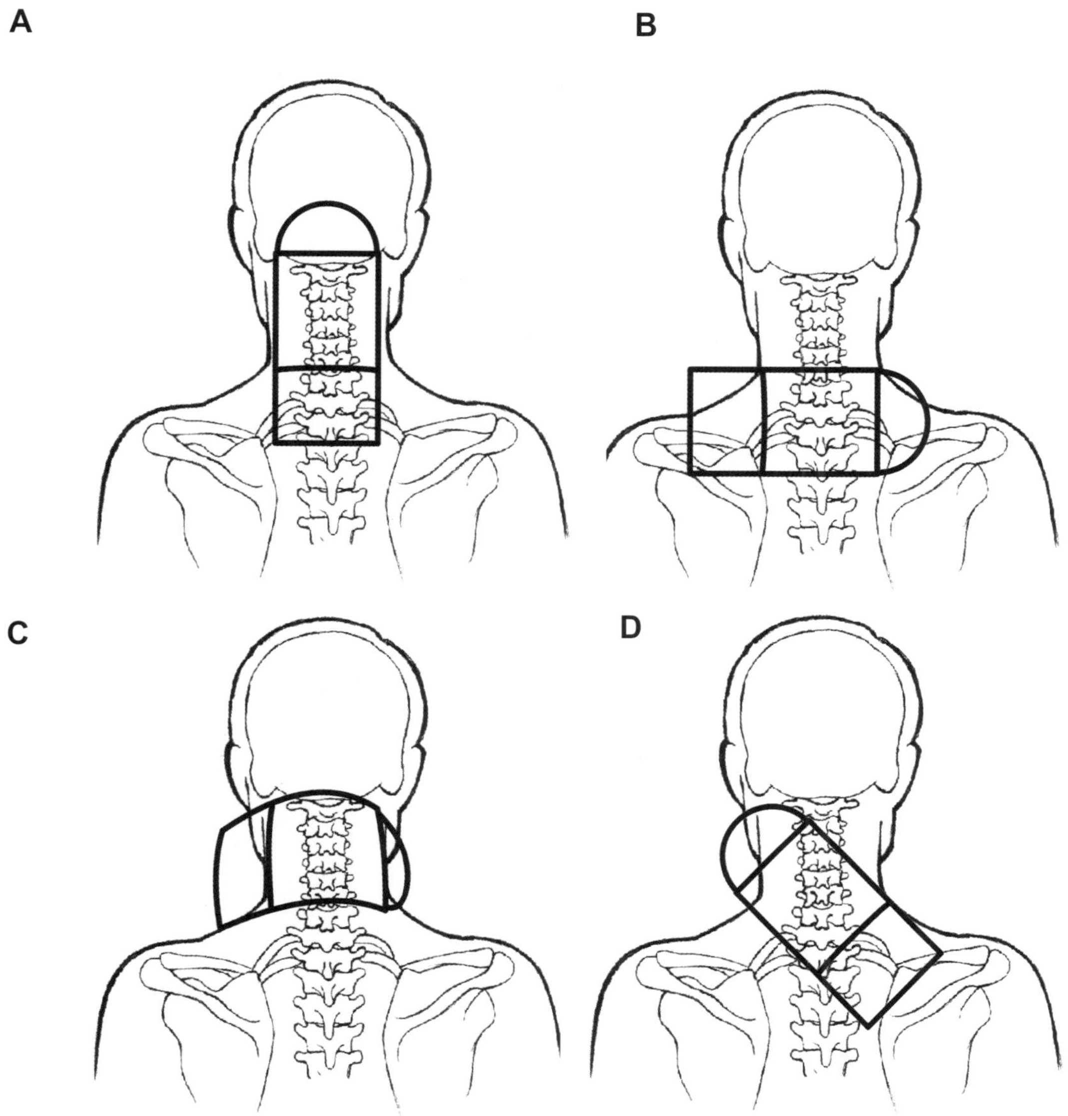

Normally utilize Large Surface Array as in figure A & B. However, anatomically, placement as in figure C may be preferable to A.

LS-R 250 and LS-I 500 mW arrays may be useful for lateral placement with severe problems.

Facial Pain

Dental Problems
- Post-maxillo-facial surgery
- Post-extraction of tooth
- Gingivitis
- Haematoma
- Auditory Conditions
- Trigeminal neuralgia
- Tinnitus
- Bells Palsy

Stage One:

Treatment Head	*Frequency*	*Duty Cycle*	*Duration (minutes)*
LS-R 750 LS-I 1500 LD-I 75	CW 10-20 CW	40-70	8 12 5-8

Stage Two:

Treatment Head	*Frequency*	*Duty Cycle*	*Duration (minutes)*
LS-R 750 LS-I 1500 LD-I 75	100 50 CW	90 70-90	8 12 5-8

Stage Three:

Treatment Head	*Frequency*	*Duty Cycle*	*Duration (minutes)*
LS-R 750 LS-I 1500 LD-I 75	500-1000 250 CW or 100	90 80 90	8 12 5-8

Treatment Tips:

1) Always use protective eye shields over the eyes.
2) With auditory problems (Meniere's Disease, Tinnitus, etc.) treat over the ear in 2 dimensions transverse and vertical or oblique and utilize the laser probe over mastoid bone and auditory canal in circumferential fashion.

Facial Pain

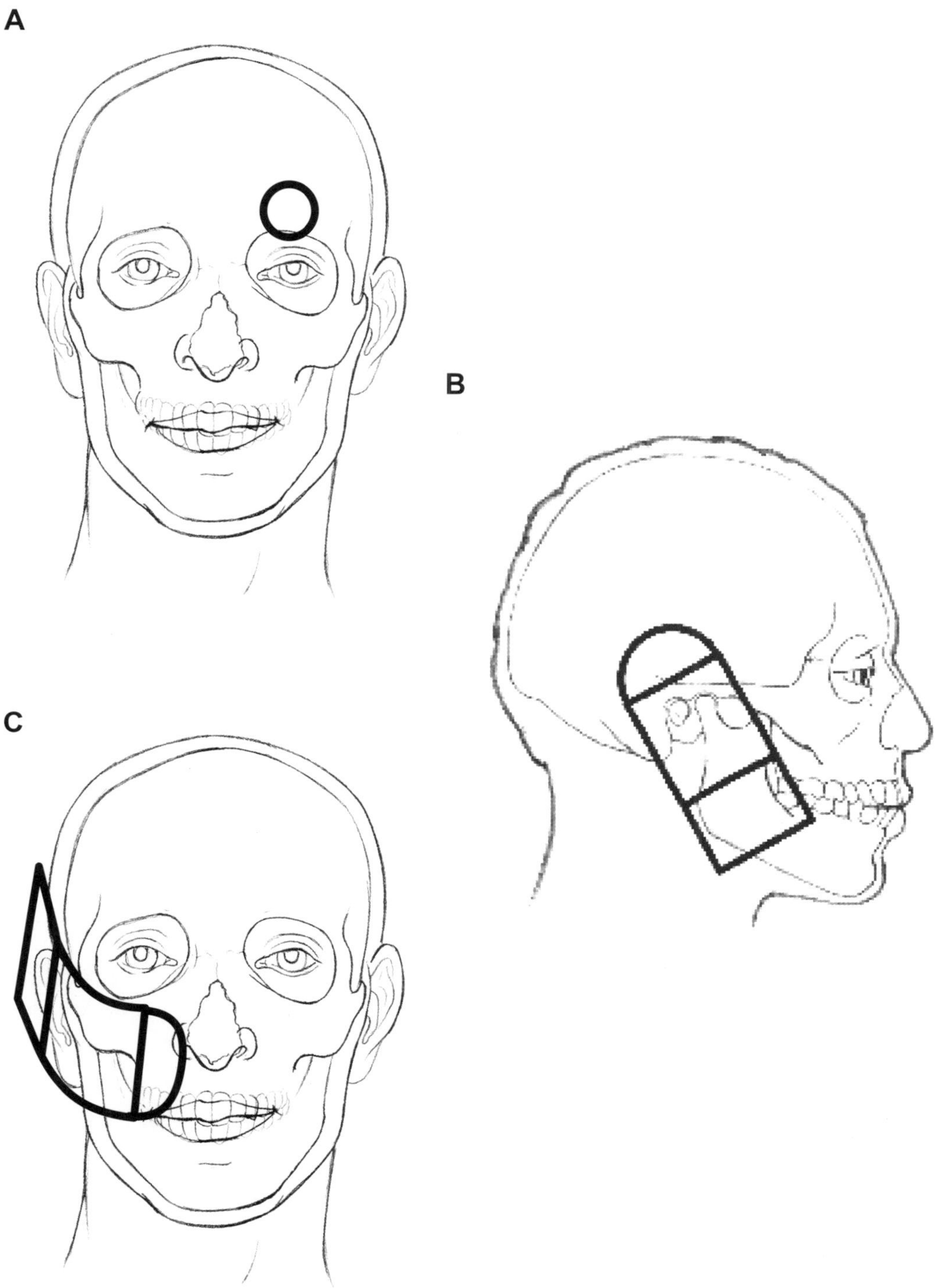

Tempero-Mandibular Joint (TMJ) Dysfunction

Stage One:

Treatment Head	*Frequency*	*Duty Cycle*	*Duration (minutes)*
LS-R 250	CW		8
LS-I 500	10-20	40-70	8
LD-I 75	CW		6

Stage Two:

Treatment Head	*Frequency*	*Duty Cycle*	*Duration (minutes)*
LS-R 250	100	80	8
LS-I 500	50	50-80	8
LD-I 75	CW		6

Stage Three:

Treatment Head	*Frequency*	*Duty Cycle*	*Duration (minutes)*
LS-R 250	250-1000	80	8
LS-I 500	50	90	8
LD-I 75	CW or 100	90	6

Treatment Tips:

1) With Tempero-Mandibular Joint Dysfunction duration of therapy may be reduced in acute conditions initially particularly if multiple additional areas are being treated. If the shorter treatment time is ineffective after several sessions return to regular mode of application.
2) For a reduced time variation for the treatment of tempero-mandibular joint apply the R-250 CW for 6 minutes, the IR-500 at a frequency of 50Hz and with a duty cycle of 80% for 6 minutes and the IR-75 laser probe for 5 minutes.

Tempero-Mandibular Joint (TMJ) Dysfunction

A

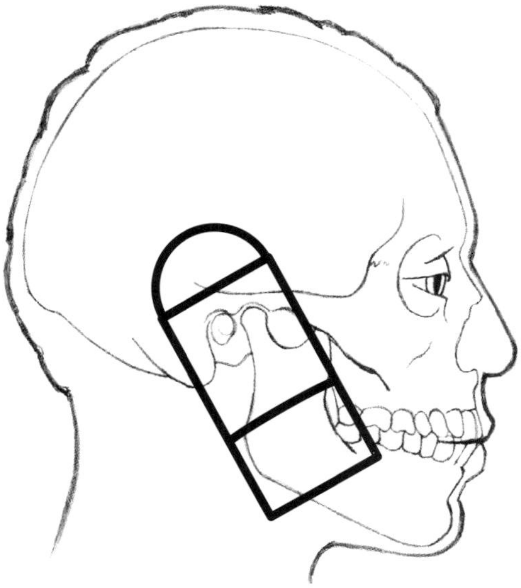

B

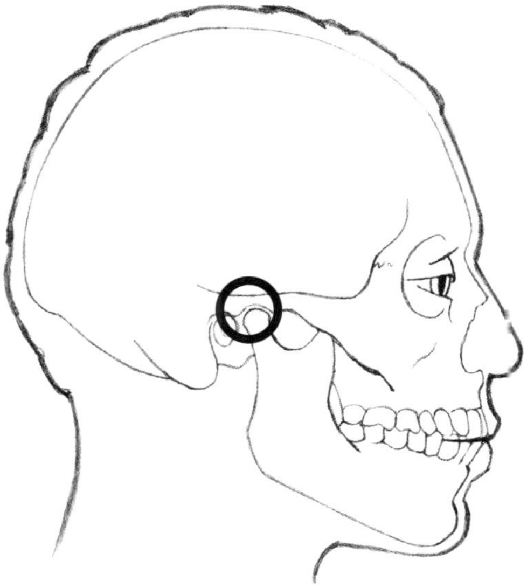

C

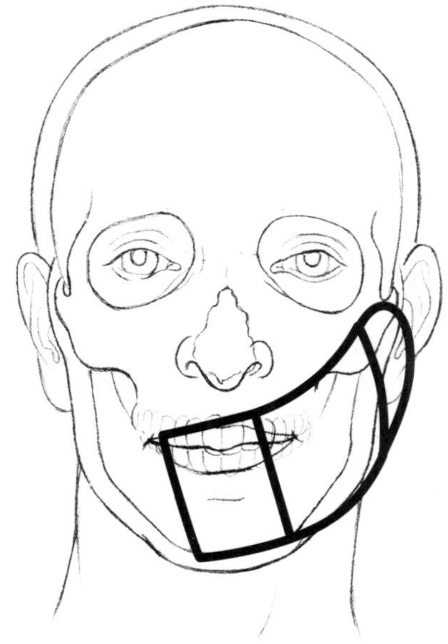

Herpes Zoster

Stage One:

Treatment Head	*Frequency*	*Duty Cycle*	*Duration (minutes)*
LS-R 750	50	50	10
LS-I 1500	10-40	60	15
LD-I 75	CW		5

Stage Two:

Treatment Head	*Frequency*	*Duty Cycle*	*Duration (minutes)*
LS-R 750	CW		10
LS-I 1500	50	70-90	15
LD-I 75	CW		5

Stage Three:

Treatment Head	*Frequency*	*Duty Cycle*	*Duration (minutes)*
LS-R 750	250-1000	90	10
LS-I 1500	250	80	15
LD-I 75	CW or 100	80	5

Treatment Tips:

1) Frequent change of protocols may be required due to viral mutation and other factors.
2) Always obtain maximum benefit of the first treatment stage prior to proceeding to the second stage.
3) May not require treatment of dermal lesions. Apply appropriate clinical judgement.
4) Remain at low levels as long as positive impact on tissues continues.

Herpes Zoster

A

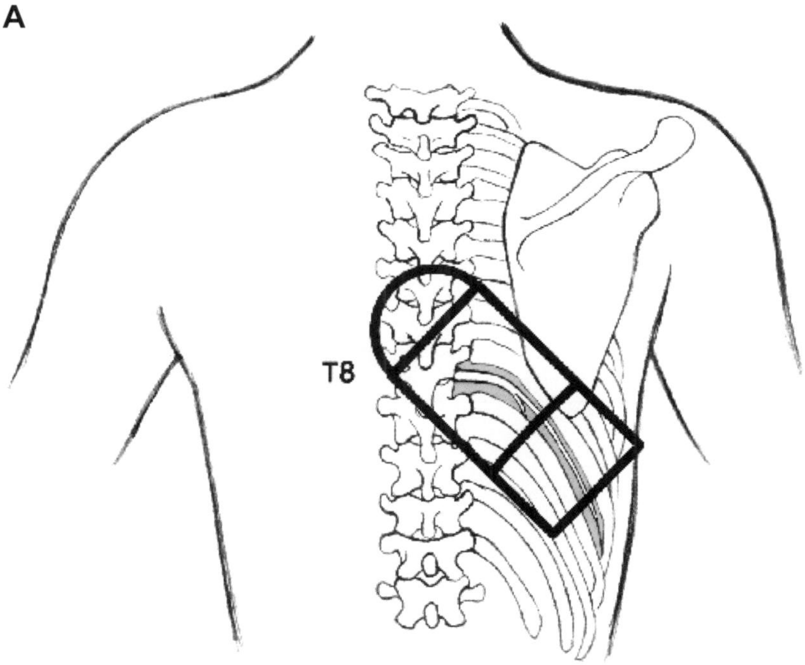

B

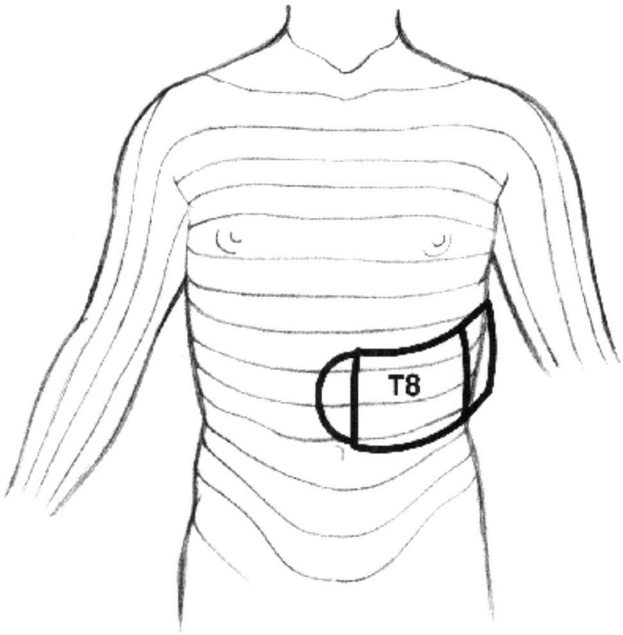

Treat nerve roots involved, at their origin and along the course of the nerve as required.

Most important to treat spinal cord and nerve roots.

Rheumatoid Arthritis

Stage One:

Treatment Head	*Frequency*	*Duty Cycle*	*Duration (minutes)*
LS-R 750	50	50	10
LS-I 1500	10	20-80	15
LD-I 75	50	50	5

Stage Two:

Treatment Head	*Frequency*	*Duty Cycle*	*Duration (minutes)*
LS-R 750	CW		10
LS-I 1500	20-50	50-90	15
LD-I 75	CW		5

Stage Three:

Treatment Head	*Frequency*	*Duty Cycle*	*Duration (minutes)*
LS-R 750	250-1000	90	10
LS-I 1500	250	80	15
LD-I 75	CW		5

Treatment Tips:

1) Applies to all areas.
2) Stage three may go to higher frequencies for LS-I 1500 as tolerated.
3) In some cases higher levels required as tissue adapts.

Lymphaedema

- Post Mastectomy - obstruction of lymph channels in the upper extremities
- Venous or lymphatic - obstructive pathology of the lower extremities
- Congenital, systemic or positional causes

Stage One:

Treatment Head	*Frequency*	*Duty Cycle*	*Duration (minutes)*
LS-R 750 LS-I 1500 LD-I 75	CW 10-50 CW	20-80	5/5 7/7 6

Stage Two:

Treatment Head	*Frequency*	*Duty Cycle*	*Duration (minutes)*
LS-R 750 LS-I 1500 LD-I 75	100 50 CW	90 50-90	5/5 7/7 6

Stage Three:

Treatment Head	*Frequency*	*Duty Cycle*	*Duration (minutes)*
LS-R 750 LS-I 1500 LD-I 75	250-1000 250 CW or 100	90 80-90 90	5/5 7/7 6

Treatment Tips:

1) Stage three may go to higher frequencies particularly with LS-I 1500.
2) Apply in series of positions, moving proximal to distal regions in sequence.
3) Probe may not be required if no major focal area.
4) Use large surface arrays in a circumferential fashion on the involved limb. Initiate treatment proximally and work distally beyond the area of edema for one to two inches. Devote a greater proportion of treatment time anteriorly or posteriorly depending on location of the major pathology, i.e. 2/3 of the treatment time to most severe area and 1/3 to the remainder of limb circumference (usually posterior aspect is most severely affected.)
5) If vascular component exists also treat the termial spinal cord.

Fibromyalgia

Stage One:

Treatment Head	*Frequency*	*Duty Cycle*	*Duration (minutes)*
LS-R 750	50	50	10
LS-I 1500	10-40	30-80	15
LD-I 75	20	30	5

Stage Two:

Treatment Head	*Frequency*	*Duty Cycle*	*Duration (minutes)*
LS-R 750	CW		10
LS-I 1500	50	50-90	15
LD-I 75	CW		5

Stage Three:

Treatment Head	*Frequency*	*Duty Cycle*	*Duration (minutes)*
LS-R 750	1000	90	10
LS-I 1500	250	80-90	15
LD-I 75	CW or 100	70-80	5

Treatment Tips:

1) Initially, treat the most severely affected areas. This will frequently resolve symptoms in less severely involved areas without treatment, as is also frequently the case in biomechanical problems.

Dermatological Applications

- Scars
- Acne
- Psoriasis

Stage One:

Treatment Head	Frequency	Duty Cycle	Duration (minutes)
LS-R 750	10 -30	50	12
LS-I 1500	50	50	12
LD-I 75	CW		6

Stage Two:

Treatment Head	Frequency	Duty Cycle	Duration (minutes)
LS-R 750	100-500	80-90	12
LS-I 1500	50	80	12
LD-I 75	CW		6

Stage Three:

Treatment Head	Frequency	Duty Cycle	Duration (minutes)
LS-R 750	1000	90	12
LS-I 1500	5000	80-90	12
LD-I 75	CW		6

Treatment Tips:

1) Flexibility is the key in these situations.
2) Additional studies are currently under way.
3) Length and size of the scars/ striae/ varicosities are factors that determine duration and frequency of treatment
4) Correlate with clinical response.
5) Persistence sometimes important.

Generic I Degenerative Osteoarthritis

Stage One:

Treatment Head	*Frequency*	*Duty Cycle*	*Duration (minutes)*
LS-R 750	CW		8
LS-I 1500	50	50-80	8/8
LD-I 75	CW		6

Stage Two:

Treatment Head	*Frequency*	*Duty Cycle*	*Duration (minutes)*
LS-R 750	CW		8
LS-I 1500	250	90	8/8
LD-I 75	CW		6

Stage Three:

Treatment Head	*Frequency*	*Duty Cycle*	*Duration (minutes)*
LS-R 750	1000	90	8
LS-I 1500	250-5000	90	8/8
LD-I 75	CW or 100	90	6 or more

Treatment Tips:

1) Unless the condition is localized, one hour of treatment is generally required, i.e. hip, lumbar and thoracic spine, and sometimes even cervical spine.

Generic II Tendonitis

Stage One:

Treatment Head	*Frequency*	*Duty Cycle*	*Duration (minutes)*
LS-R 750	50	50	10
LS-I 1500	10	20-60	15
LD-I 75	CW		5

Stage Two:

Treatment Head	*Frequency*	*Duty Cycle*	*Duration (minutes)*
LS-R 750	100	50-90	10
LS-I 1500	20	40-80	15
LD-I 75	CW		5

Stage Three:

Treatment Head	*Frequency*	*Duty Cycle*	*Duration (minutes)*
LS-R 750	250	70-90	10
LS-I 1500	250	80-90	15
LD-I 75	CW or 100	70-90	5

Generic III Inflammatory Conditions

Stage One:

Treatment Head	*Frequency*	*Duty Cycle*	*Duration (minutes)*
LS-R 750	50	50	8/8
LS-I 1500	10-40	30-70	8/8
LD-I 75	CW		6

Stage Two:

Treatment Head	*Frequency*	*Duty Cycle*	*Duration (minutes)*
LS-R 750	CW		8/8
LS-I 1500	50	40-80	8/8
LD-I 75	CW		6

Stage Three:

Treatment Head	*Frequency*	*Duty Cycle*	*Duration (minutes)*
LS-R 750	250-1000	90	8/8
LS-I 1500	250	80-90	8/8
LD-I 75	CW or 100	70-90	6

Treatment Tips:

1) Generally stage one is adequate with the duration ranging from 30-60 minutes depending on the extent of the pathology.

Generic IV Autoimmune Conditions

Stage One:

Treatment Head	*Frequency*	*Duty Cycle*	*Duration (minutes)*
LS-R 750	20	40	10
LS-I 1500	10	20	14
LD-I 75	50	50	6

Stage Two:

Treatment Head	*Frequency*	*Duty Cycle*	*Duration (minutes)*
LS-R 750	50	50	10
LS-I 1500	20	40-80	14
LD-I 75	CW		6

Stage Three:

Treatment Head	*Frequency*	*Duty Cycle*	*Duration (minutes)*
LS-R 750	100	90	10
LS-I 1500	50	50-90	14
LD-I 75	CW		6

Treatment Tips:

1) Assess frequently and direct protocols accordingly.

III Index of Conditions Treated

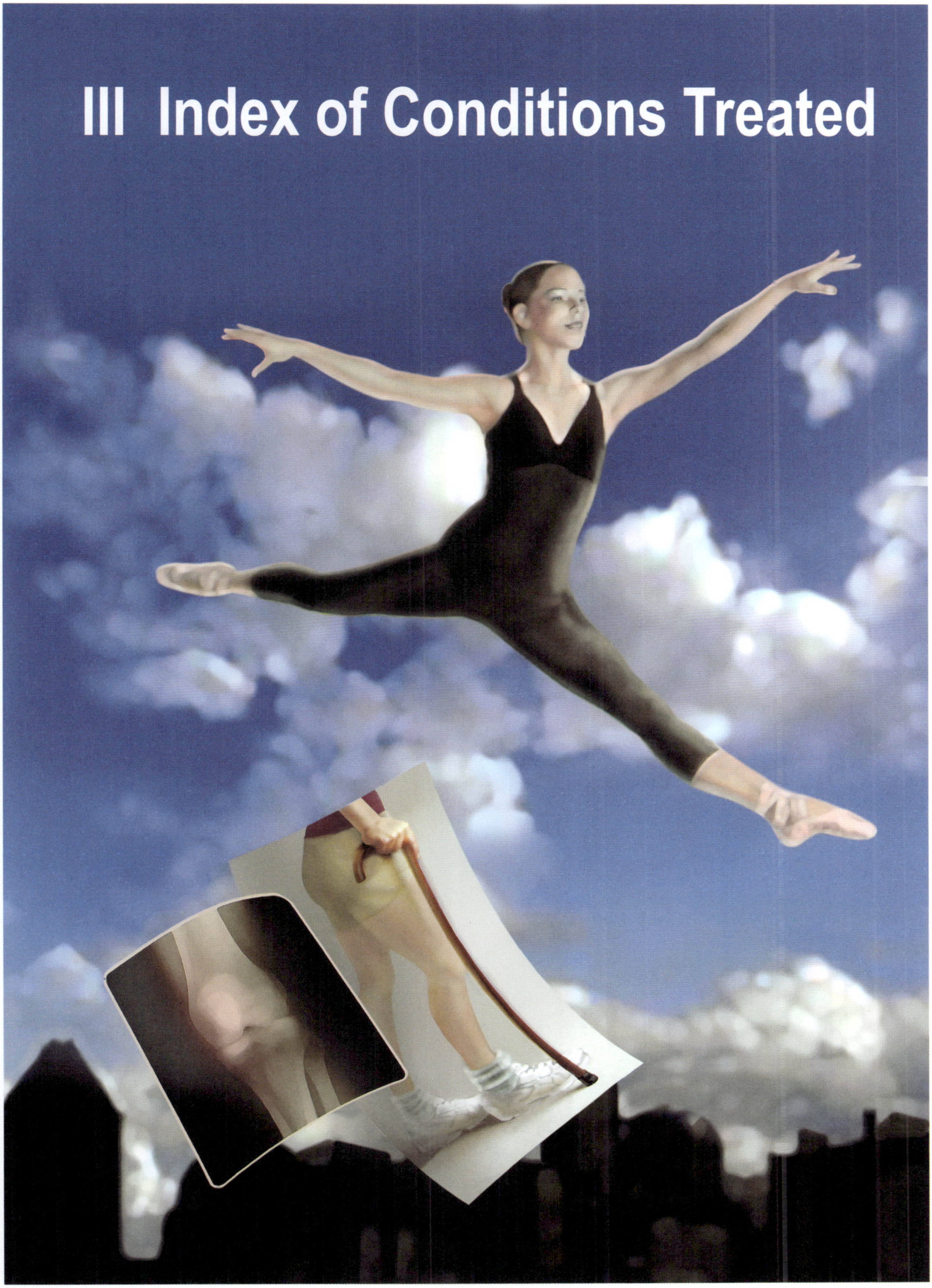

Index of Conditions Treated

IV Appendix

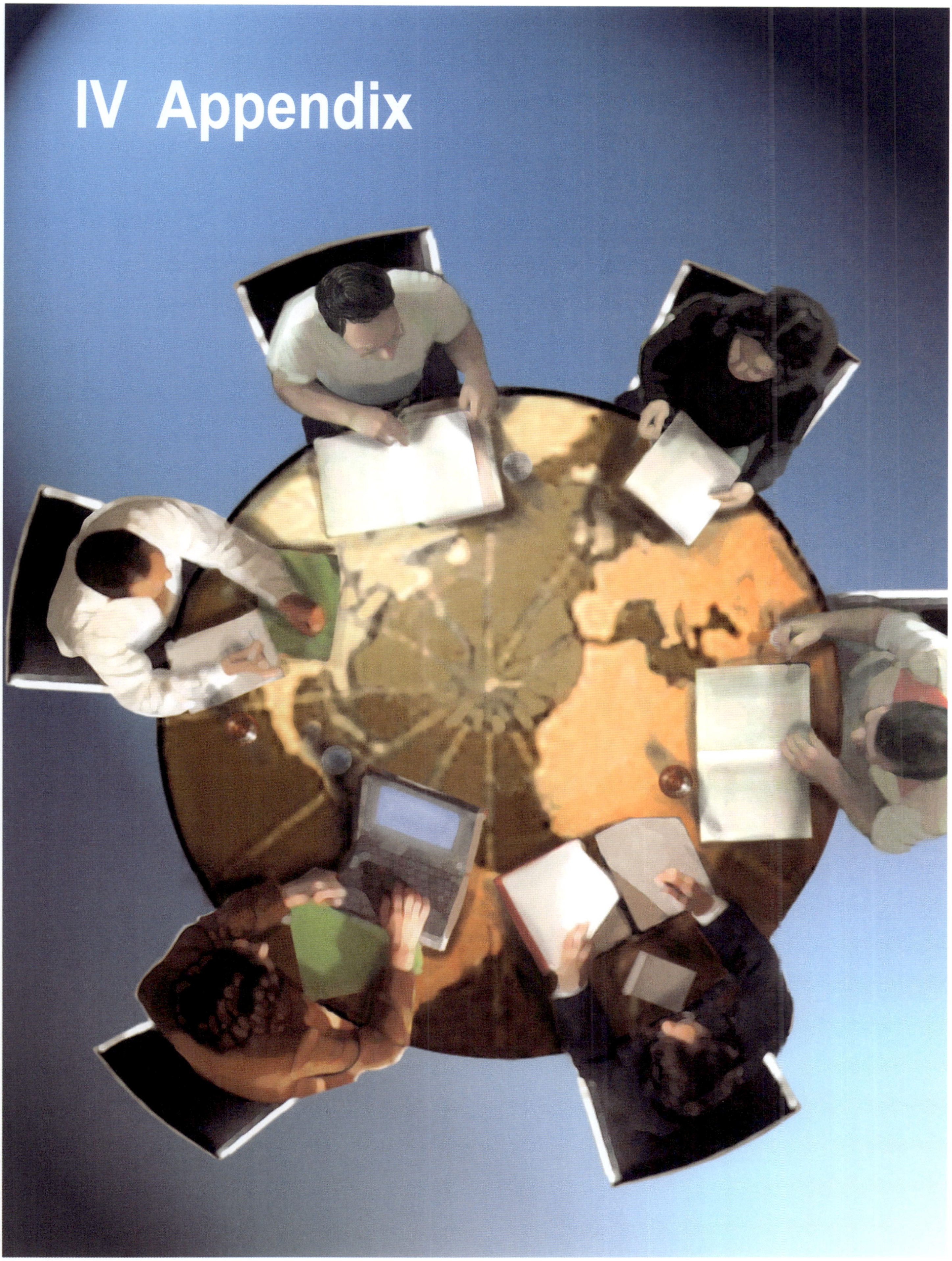

Mission Statement

Meditech International Inc. initiated research in the development of Low Intensity Laser Therapy Systems in 1988.

The goal of the company has been to engineer devices that are superior to those in existence and scientifically develop accurate, effective protocols to treat a variety of medical conditions in the musculo-skeletal field. These include sports injuries, repetitive motion syndrome and the arthritides.

To date, we have surpassed our initial goals and expectations but each day advances our horizons as the educational process continues.

Our primary objectives are to significantly improve/cure the multiple pathologies that we encounter in the shortest possible period of time. Guidelines to that end consist of the elimination of pharmaceuticals, pain and restoration of mobility and the quality of life.

Low Intensity Laser Therapy: The Clinical Approach

ABSTRACT

Recently, there has been significant improvement in the process of research and application of Low Intensity Laser Therapy (LILT). The clinical results presented in this paper are extrapolated from a wide range of musculoskeletal problems including degenerative osteoarthritis, sports injuries, etc. This paper includes three separate clinical studies comprising 151, 286 and 576 consecutive patient discharges at our clinic. The essentials of the treatment involved a photon stream emanating from a number of specified gallium-aluminum-arsenide diodes; stage one, red light array, stage two consisting of an array of infrared diodes and stage three consisting of the application of an infrared laser diode probe. On average, each of these groups required less than 10 treatments per patient and resulted in a significant improvement rate greater than 90% in all conditions treated. This report clearly demonstrates the benefits of LILT, indicating that it should be more widely adapted in medical therapeutic settings.

Keywords: Low intensity laser therapy, clinical, mobility, rehabilitation, treatment, pain reduction

INTRODUCTION

Low Intensity Laser Therapy (LILT), from both the clinical and research perspective has been scrutinized intensively during the course of its application over the past 30 years. Despite this extensive history, the utilization of lasers to heal tissue is a relatively new endeavor, particularly in North America. There are many reasons contributing to this situation:

- Lack of interest, as a preponderance of medical practice is based on the utilization of pharmaceuticals and surgical interventions.
- The majority of research papers and other publications emanate from Russian, Japanese and Eastern European laboratories, with minimal exposure in the western industrialized nations.
- Slow approval by regulatory bodies
- Non inclusion by today's gatekeepers i.e. HMO's, insurance companies, governments, etc.
- No inclusion in curriculum of educational institutions

This has resulted in a lack of acceptance by mainstream medicine which demands that more controlled double blind studies be carried out. The concept of curing pathologies with laser therapy has not fully made its impact in the practice of medicine. The majority of pharmaceuticals are not designed to heal the pathology but rather to modulate or mask symptoms. In contradistinction, LILT is designed to cure the pathology rather than to suppress symptoms.

Over the past three decades, many research groups have attempted to define the exact interaction between light and cells both in vivo and in vitro, including cell cultures of both the human and animal variety. A recent review of the literature comprising over 300 cited articles and abstracts attests to this fact. The majority of double blind clinical trials reveal an overwhelming amount of evidence supporting the positive effects achieved using LILT. Articles that are negative have generally failed in their approach owing to the use of poorly designed devices and the improper application of therapy. This includes lack of standardization, inadequate power, insufficient duration of treatment and utilizing inappropriate protocols. Furthermore, most devices in the marketplace today are deficient in design, protocols are frequently selected at random and therapists are not provided with the proper education to operate the equipment. Moreover they generally lack a basic understanding of physiology, anatomy and physics. Academics over the past decade have continued to promote additional double blind clinical trials and this is certainly commendable; in actual fact however, minimal practical progress has been achieved from the clinical perspective.

The effectiveness of laser therapy has been much debated regarding the analysis of parameters (frequency, duty cycle, waveform, etc.), environmental setting, the accuracy of the pre-therapeutic diagnosis and numerous other factors. At Meditech, we recognized these problems 15 years ago at the inception of our research and this publication shares some observations in addition to the results achieved with our new clinical approach to healing.

METHODS

The outcomes in these studies are derived from the utilization of therapy delivered by the BioFlex Professional System manufactured by Meditech International Incorporated. This system was developed over the course of 16 years by a group headed by Dr. Fred Kahn. Over the course of time, valuable contributions were made by Professor Tiina Karu, Dr. Mary Dyson, numerous clinicians and the Engineering Department at Ryerson University in Toronto. Initially, 20 systems were developed for proof of concept purposes. The current system has been in operation in a clinical setting at Meditech's Treatment Centres and at numerous independent clinics in 22 countries throughout the world. Patients in our studies were carefully diagnosed by a small number of medical specialists and treatments were prescribed on the basis of Meditech's Clinical Users Manual directives and customized as clinically indicated. All therapeutic procedures were carried out in uniform fashion based on a combination of accurate diagnosis, clinical experience and the utililization of the correct protocols. Consistency was the keynote throughout the entire process. Changes in treatment procedure were based on clinical progress both positive and negative on each individual patient visit. In 70% of all patients treated, the protocols utilized were standard and customization was carried out in the additional 30%. This consistent methodology is felt to be essential in the achievement of superior clinical outcomes.

Primary objectives of the treatment were:

1. Elimination of pain.
2. Substantial increase in mobility and range of motion.
3. Cessation of the utilization of multiple medications (analgesics, NSAIDs and cortisone.)
4. Improvement of the patient's overall status (normal sleep patterns, activity levels, appetite and headache relief, etc.)
5. To enable the patient to resume normal work patterns and physical activities.

To reach these goals required an intense effort and close collaboration between the patient, physician and the therapist applying the treatment. This attention to detail is essential to the achievement of positive results in the preponderance of patients, the objective in all instances being a total cure.

Invariably the treatment regime utilized in these studies consisted of the three stage approach. Super luminous diode arrays and lasers from 660 to 840 nm wavelength were employed in individual arrays. In certain circles the debate of utilizing laser versus superluminous diodes remains controversial and we adhere to the dictum that the results speak for themselves. The major difference between these two types of light remains coherence. In the treatment of biological tissue this coherence is lost within the first 5 to 10 µm as it is differentially scattered. This clearly supports the use of superluminous diodes as being equally efficient in the treatment of cells. The singular advantage of using laser diodes is that the power output is generated in a confined area resulting in deeper penetration, useful in treating the primary focus of any pathology. The three stage approach that we utilize covers a wide range of varying penetration depths and chromophore absorption. The stages are delivered using the following arrays:

1. Red light (660 nm) using a 180 diode array of superluminous diodes.
2. Infrared light (840 nm) using a 180 diode array of superluminous diodes.
3. Infrared laser probe (830 nm) using a single laser source focused on the basic pathology.

Low Intensity Laser Therapy was utilized as the basic platform in the therapeutic program which was augmented in approximately 50% of cases by massage, thermal therapy and at the later stage exercise programmes. These are therapies that we use to speed up the process initially, particularly in acute and extensive injuries but were not felt to be essential to the treatment program.

It should be noted that over 60% of cases suffered from more than one medical problem and the majority of patients had undergone therapy varying from a matter of weeks to years under the direction of the family physician, physiotherapist, chiropractor, neurologist, rheumatologist, orthopedic surgeon or psychologist. Analgesics, anti-inflammatory medications and cortisone had been utilized extensively in the majority of the patient population and many surgical procedures had been carried out often with results that were less than desirable. It is not uncommon for a patient presenting at our clinic to indulge in the ingestion of over 30 analgesics on a daily basis. In our practice most pain can be explained applying the standard medical approach. We listen to the patient, perform a complete physical examination and utilize test procedures as indicated. Once this process has been completed, we initiate therapy, generally on the initial visit.

In all studies, a patient questionnaire was used to determine the percentage of improvement on discharge. This included a visual analogue pain scale ranging from 0 (no pain) to 10 (intolerable pain). This is seen in Figure 1.1.

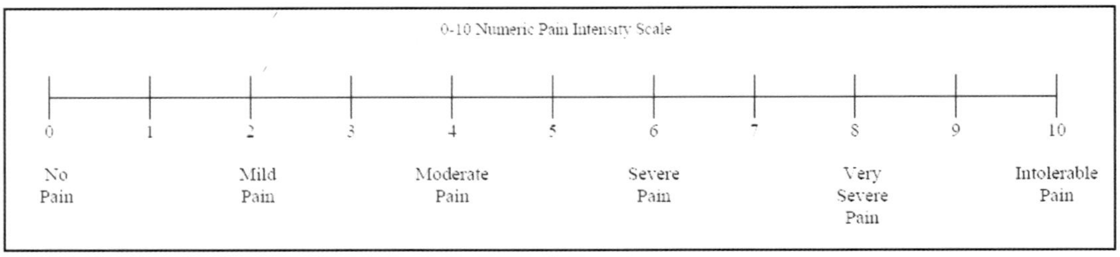

This was followed by asking the patient to state the degree of overall improvement and was based on a scale from 0% (no improvement) to 100% (complete elimination of symptoms). The numbers of these questions were then averaged into five groups and are presented as a mean ± standard deviation. The groups consisted of degenerative pathologies, repetitive strain injuries, trauma, sports injuries and other pathologies that do not conform to the previous categories.

The following three sections are the separate clinical studies, comprised of 151, 286 and 576 patients. Each section contains both a summary of the patients treated as well as the results from the questionnaire that was competed at the last treatment session.

STUDY ONE

Patients:

One hundred and fifty-one patients (n=151); consisting of ninety-four males (n=94) and fifty-seven females (n=57) participated in the first clinical study. The average age of the patients was forty-six years (age=46±12 years). Separating the patients into distinct pathology groups resulted in 29% of the patients falling into the category of degenerative osteoarthritis. The majority of these involved the lumbo-sacral spine and over 60% of these were accompanied by degenerative disc disease, bulging discs, nerve root compression and/ or stenosis of the spinal canal or foramen. The percentage of different pathologies treated in this study can be seen in Figure 2.1.

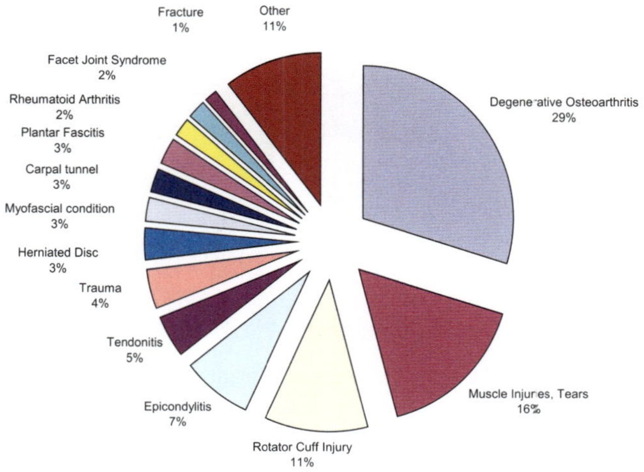

Figure 2.1. The percentage of each condition treated in the first study.

Results:

The results of the first clinical study were that patients had a 90.4% improvement over an average of 11 treatments. The average visual analog pain scale rating was 0.22 out of 10. The overall improvements for the different pathologies are presented in Table 1.

Table 1. Percentage improvement and average number of treatments for the different pathologies treated in the first clinical study

Condition	Number of Patients	Average number of treatments	Percentage overall improvement
Degenerative	48	12.6	86.3
Repetitive Stress Injury	28	11.5	87.8
Trauma	36	10.7	95.6
Sports Injury	22	9.3	94.4
Other	17	11.2	90
Mean ± Standard Deviation	151	11.3 ± 1.0	90.4 ± 6.8

Discussion:

The results of this study are encouraging in the treatment of a range of pathologies with LILT. Further improvement of protocols throughout this study revealed a diminishing number of treatments and increased the overall improvement of the patients. This trend should continue as both the treatment experience and the refinement of protocols expand.

One patient particularly highlights the success in treating a variety of pathologies using LILT. The patient was an 86 year old podiatrist who had periphero-arterial occlusive disease that created a pre-gangrenous status in his feet. The problem had been complicated by severe frostbite of his toes during a prior skiing excursion. He was advised that partial amputation would be necessary. The patient decided to find alternative therapy and presented at our clinic. The first picture (Figure 2.2a) was taken on arrival prior to his first treatment; 6 months after he had initial symptoms in the foot.

a) b)

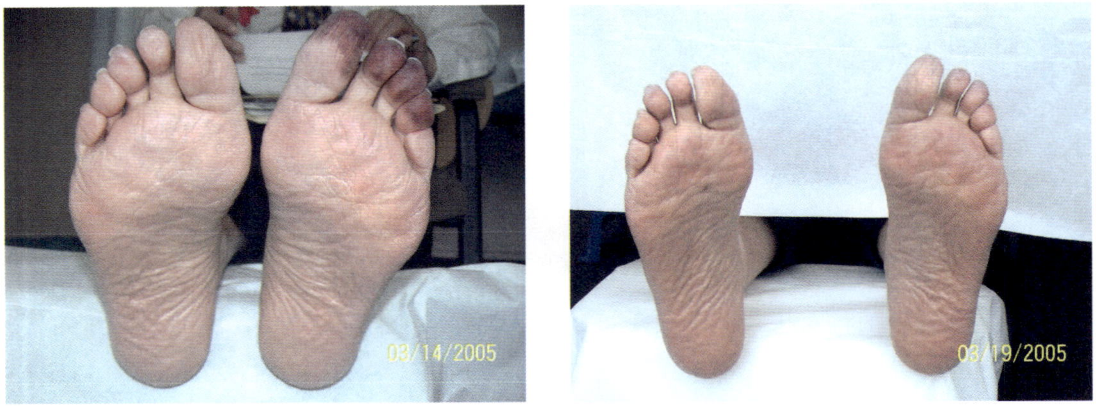

Figure 2.2 a) The initial picture before any treatment with LILT.

b) The final picture after 5 consecutive days of treatment with LILT.

After the first treatment he noted a reduction in pain and an increase in the temperature of the foot. Treatments were 60 minutes in duration and were administered daily for five days both locally and over the spinal cord and sympathetic ganglia. The improvement in temperature continued throughout the treatment and by the fifth day it had returned to normal; the pain and discoloration were completely gone (Figure 2.2b). The toes had regained normal function.

STUDY TWO

Patients:

Two hundred and eighty-six patients (n=286); consisting of one hundred and seventy males (n=170) and one hundred and sixteen females (n=116) participated in the second clinical study. The average age of the patients was fifty-three years (age=53±17 years). Separating the patients into distinct pathology groups resulted in 46% of the patients falling into the category of degenerative osteoarthritis, which is 17% higher than the first study. The segmentation of pathologies can be seen in Figure 3.1.

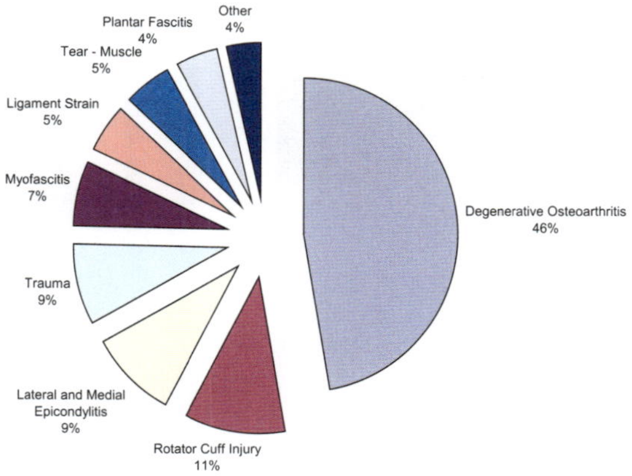

Figure 3.1 The percentage of each condition treated in the second study.

Results:

The results of this clinical study were that patients had a 91.1% improvement over an average of 9.7 treatments for all conditions. The average visual analog pain scale rating was 0.19 out of 10. The improvements for the different pathologies are presented in Table 2.

Table 2. Percentage improvement and average number of treatments for the different pathologies treated in the second clinical study.

Condition	Number of Patients	Average number of treatments	Percentage overall improvement
Degenerative	108	11.5	87.6
Repetitive Stress Injury	35	10.7	88.7
Trauma	48	8.9	93
Sports Injury	89	7.8	96
Other	6	11.1	91.1
Mean ± Standard Deviation	286	9.7 ± 0.96	91.1 ± 6.84

Discussion:

The results from this study show an improvement over the first study containing 151 patients. This improvement can be attributed to better knowledge including improved protocol selection, application and experience.

As the patient load increases, we note a commensurate increase in the number of back problems, degenerative arthritis, and sports injuries. Our surveys indicate that this is based on patient and physician referrals, the result of superior treatment outcomes. Moreover the athletes treated, both at the high performance amateur and professional level, are highly motivated to return to activity. This group has developed a dependence on this dramatic therapeutic approach to return them to action more quickly than conventional therapies. The majority of these sports injuries consist of trauma to muscles, tendons, ligaments and bone structures.

An example of these sports injuries is an athlete who had a partial tear of the left Achilles tendon. This resulted in the inability to plantar flex the foot as it was exceedingly painful (Figure 3.2a). The edema around the tendon is quite obvious and left untreated would heal with scar tissue formation and possible functional impairment. Incidentally this patient had rejected treatment of six weeks in a cast offered by her orthopedic surgeon, a customary method of therapy.

a) b)

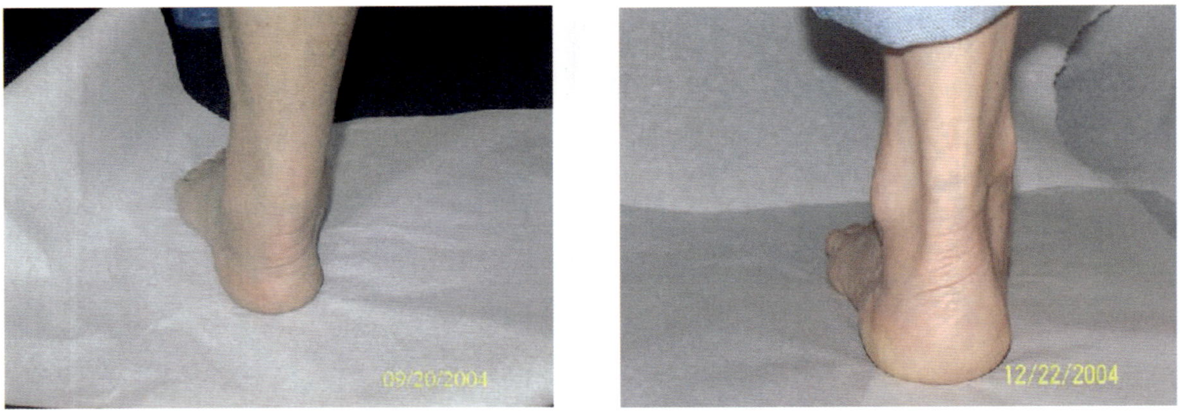

Figure 3.2 a) The initial picture before any treatment with LILT.

b) The final picture after 10 treatments over 3 months.

The superficial nature of the Achilles tendon makes it easy to treat. This patient received 10 treatments over 5 weeks and was able to return to competition. The reduction in the edema around the tendon is clearly evident (Figure 3.2b). At the end of the treatment the strength of the tendon had returned to normal accompanied by full function.

Once again, one can only state that Low Intensity Laser Therapy judiciously applied produces results unequaled by other technologies if the appropriate criteria are observed. Furthermore, it reinforces the fact that LILT is the therapy of choice in the treatment of musculoskeletal pathologies.

STUDY THREE

Patients:

Five hundred and seventy-six patients (n=576); comprised of three hundred and seventeen males (n=317) and two hundred and fifty-nine females (n=259) participated in the third clinical study. The average age of the patients was fifty-three years (age=53±16 years). The range of pathologies treated and the rate of occurrence can be seen in Figure 4.1.

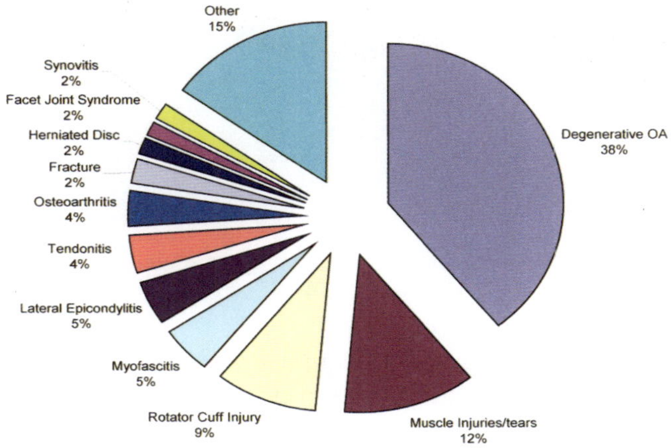

Figure 4.1. The percentage of each condition treated in the third study.

Results:

The results of the third clinical study were that patients had a 93.6% improvement over an average of 9.7 treatments for all conditions. The average visual analog pain scale rating was 0.16 out of 10. The improvements for the different pathologies are presented in Table 3.

Table 3. Percentage improvement and average number of treatments for the different pathologies treated in the third clinical study.

Condition	Number of Patients	Average number of treatments	Percentage overall improvement
Degenerative	140	11.3	88.3
Repetitive Stress Injury	93	9.6	94.3
Trauma	66	9.4	936
Sports Injury	258	9.2	96.1
Other	19	7.5	96.3
Mean ± Standard Deviation	576	9.7 ± 0.96	93.6 ± 6.84

Discussion:

The results from the third study show an improvement over the first two clinical studies containing 151 patients and 286 patients respectively. Again, there was an improvement in the cure rate as well as a reduction in the average number of treatments when compared with the two previous studies.

Throughout this study we continued to treat a number of chronic ulcers; the majority of these had existed over 6 months. The treatment of ulcers has been very challenging as the continued application of ointments, creams and dressings often increases the size of the ulcer. LILT when properly applied has an immense ability to heal lesions that would otherwise progress to more serious complications. An example of this was a patient who had thrombophlebitis of the left lower leg and multiple dermal ulcers of both extremities. This condition had been present for 14 months and the patient had been hospitalized for 3 months without improvement. He discharged himself from hospital against medical advice. The leg was in jeopardy and clearly in danger of requiring amputation (Figure 4.2).

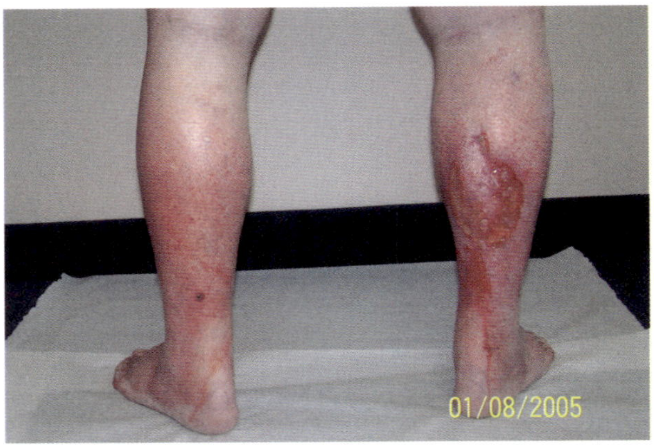

Figure 4.2. At the initial assessment the right leg has a large ulcer.

Prior to the initial treatment the diameter of the right calf was 6 cm greater than the left secondary to thrombophlebitis. The patient had 48 treatments over a period of 3 months owing to the severity of the condition and as it had been present for over 14 months before commencing LILT. The patient was placed on a regime of warm saline compresses, laser treatment on alternate days and the wounds were left open. His compliance with the outlined treatment was less than ideal. When the patient arrived he was unable to walk and had extreme pain suppressed by large quantities of analgesics. He was also on massive doses of a variety of antibiotics. Antibiotics were discontinued at the beginning of laser therapy and wounds were treated by open exposure. At the termination of his treatment (Figure 4.3) he was able to walk and had ceased to take any medications as he was pain free.

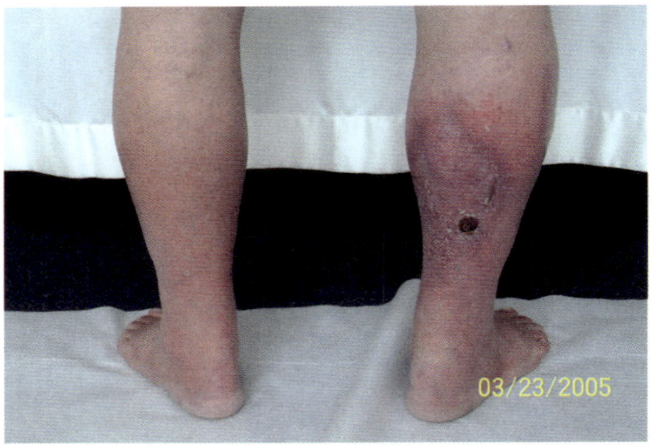

Figure 4.3. Near the final treatment the ulcer has fully healed over and the thrombophlebitis has been resolved.

A second patient in this study presented another therapeutic challenge. A 16 year old national caliber tennis player, who was riding his bike, caught the tire in the space between the sidewalk and the grass and was catapulted over the handle bars at high speed. This young man sustained spinal cord shock and a tear to the right brachial plexus. This injury was a serious threat to his tennis career as he was unable to move his arm. The initial assessment demonstrated severe loss of motor function of the muscles of the neck and of the right arm (Figure 4.4).

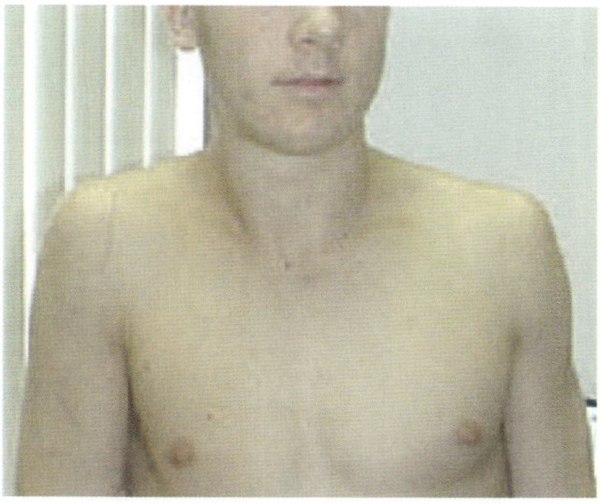

Figure 4.4. At the initial assessment the patient was unable to move his right arm and had limited movement of the neck.

He had extensive neurological work up at a major university hospital but no solutions were offered; moreover no improvement had occurred over a 4 week period prior to treatment with LILT. After the initial treatments, he gradually began to recover motor function (Figure 4.5).

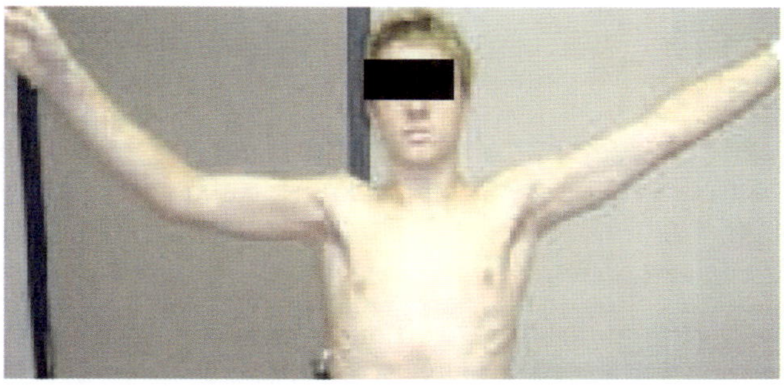

Figure 4.5. Halfway through treatment there was obvious improvement in the range of motion. The neck has resumed a more midline position. The abduction of the right are

The treatment continued over 8 weeks during which he received 15 one hour treatment sessions to the cervical spine and brachial plexus. LILT was augmented with massage therapy to help accelerate the healing process. At the completion of treatment he had regained complete power of the muscles along with a full range of motion of the arm and neck (Figure 4.6).

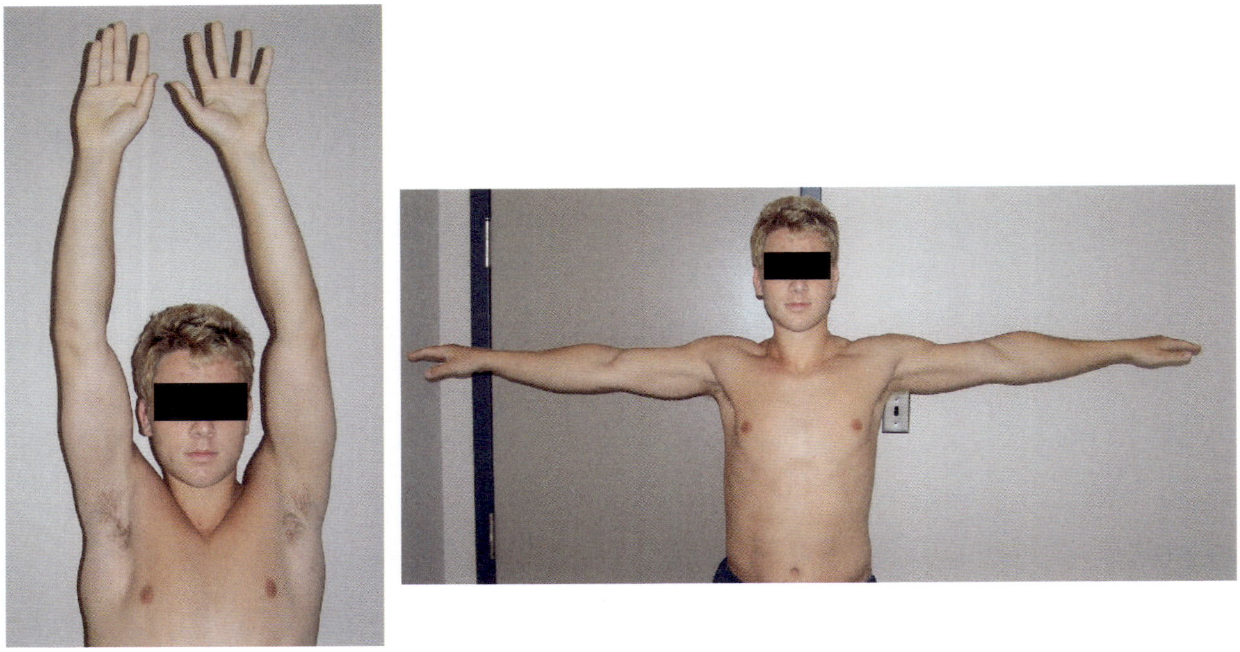

Figure 4.6. At the end of the treatment there is a full recovery with a normal range of motion.

Moreover he was able to accept a full tennis scholarship. This demonstrates the effectiveness of LILT in treating a wide range of conditions that might have otherwise been difficult to resolve.

CONCLUSION AND DISCUSSION

In these three studies we have demonstrated the effectiveness of treating a broad range of musculoskeletal pathologies with Low Intensity Laser Therapy. Each study revealed an improved cure rate with a concomitant reduction in the number of treatments required. This is clear evidence of the refinement of treatment protocol selection and application.

The four patients presented can be characterized as problematic therapeutic challenges and are a testimonial to the healing potential of Low Intensity Laser Therapy. Moreover, they should provide a stimulus to future research to enhance the understanding of the technology and its wider application.

The Clinical Presentation

Dr. Kahn has delivered this continually evolving presentation on many occasions over the last eight years in order to advance and stimulate the educational process and the knowledge base of the medical community. It has been presented at conferences and for medical professionals attending the Laser Therapy Certification Program on a regular basis.

This lecture relates to Low Intensity Laser Therapy on a conceptual basis and reflects Dr. Kahn's doctrine of: "Res Ipsa Loquitor", i.e. let the results speak for themselves.

Leslie C Perrin
Meditech International

1.

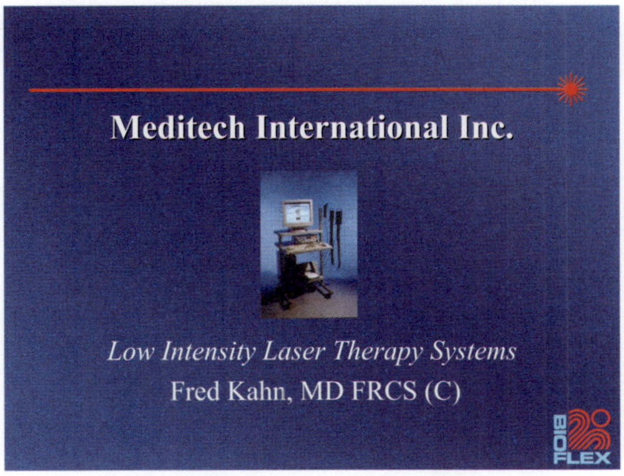

2.

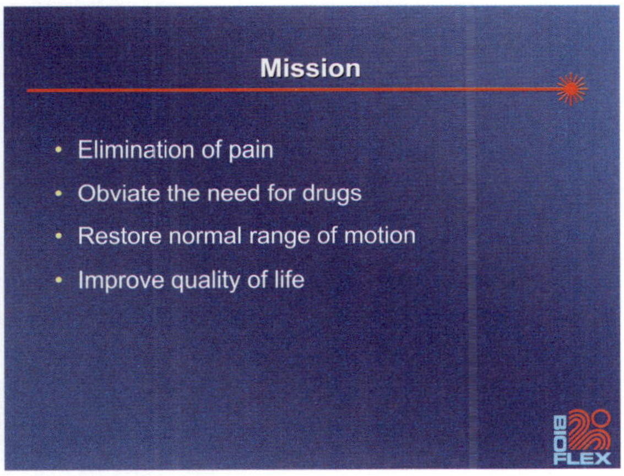

3.

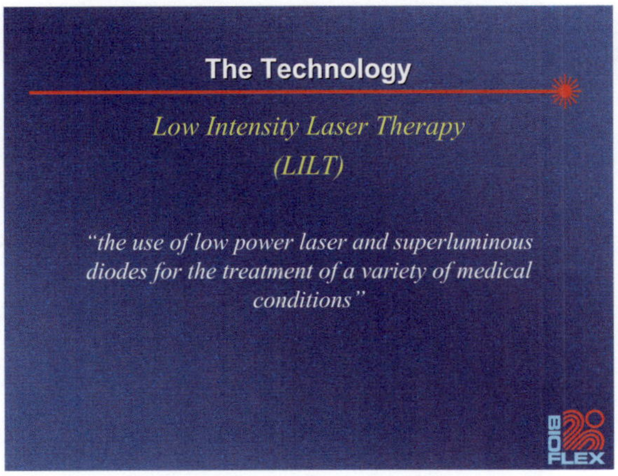

4.

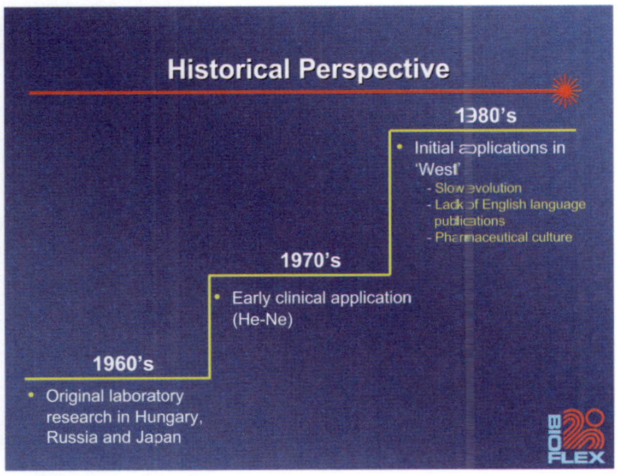

5.

Meditech's Leap into the 21st Century

- Large Surface Flexible Arrays
- Scientifically developed & clinically tested protocols
- Ability to customize protocols
- Computerized function
- New and elegant approach to healing

BIOFLEX

6.

What is the difference in terminology?

- Laser Therapy
- Low Level Laser Therapy (LLLT)
- Low Energy Laser Therapy (LELT)
- Low Energy Photon Therapy (LEPT)
- Cold Laser Therapy
- Laser Photo biostimulation ('Biostim')

BIOFLEX

7.

Re-newed Interest in LILT

- Stimulated by improvements in technology
- Availability of better engineered variable power diodes
- Understanding and control of treatment parameters
- Increased volume of quality publications
- Laboratory and clinical studies

BIOFLEX

8.

Advantages of Laser Therapy

- Non-toxic
- Non invasive
- Ease of application
- No 'side effects'
- "Safe"
- Cost effective
- Superior alternative to
  - analgesics
  - NSAID's
  - other medications
- Obviate need for surgery
- Promotes rapid healing

BIOFLEX

9.

Mechanisms of Action

Light is absorbed by irradiated tissue
- variety of chromophores, flavoproteins and other micromolecules absorb photons
- light energy is transformed into biochemical energy
- restoration of normal cellular configuration & function

Clinical results of treatment
- reduction in pain
- subjective changes
- objective changes
- acceleration of the healing process

BIOFLEX

10.

Mechanisms of Action – Continued

Visualization of Effects
- regeneration of epithelial layer with rapid closure of wounds
- Re-establishing continuity of muscle and tendon matrix

BIOFLEX

11.

Some Interactions between Light and Cell

Red light
- affects a variety of cell types
- absorbed by the mitochondrial cytochromes present in living cells

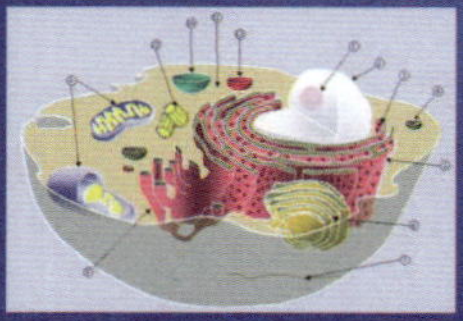

Infrared light (IR)
- absorbed by specific proteins in the cell membrane & affects permeability directly

BIOFLEX

12.

Additional Effects of Light on Cells

Mechanisms
- Temporary increase in permeability of the cell membrane to: Ca^{++}, K^{+}, Cl^{-}, Na^{+} ions
- Specific cells stimulated according to their cell type: mast cells, macrophages

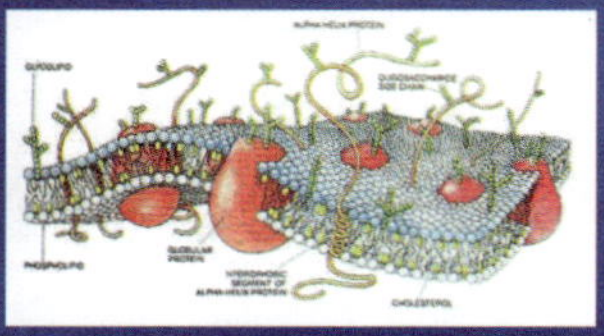

BIOFLEX

13.

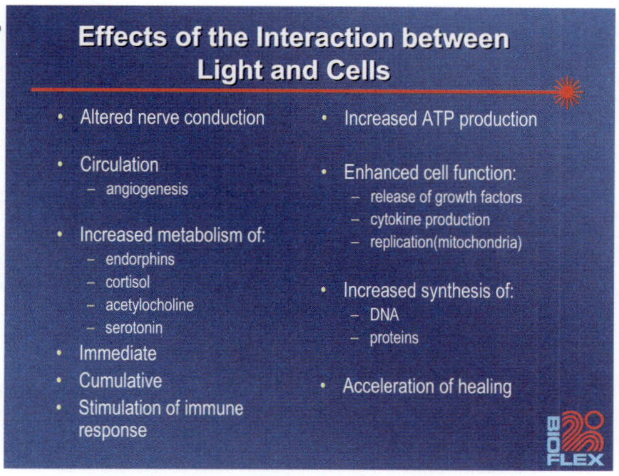

14.

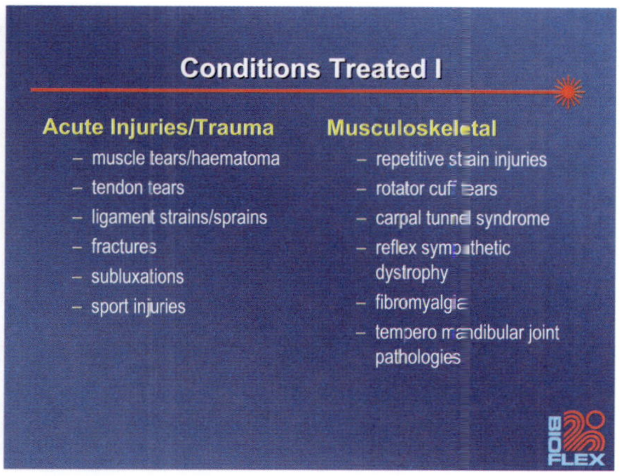

15.

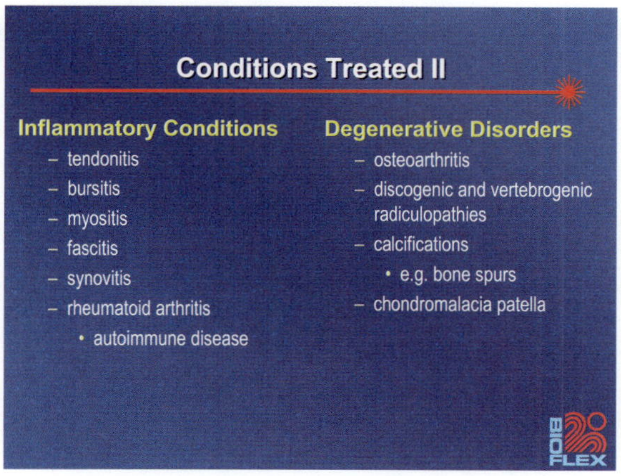

16.

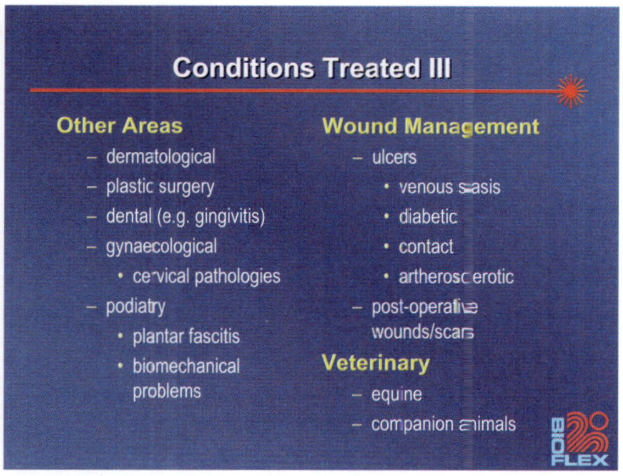

17.

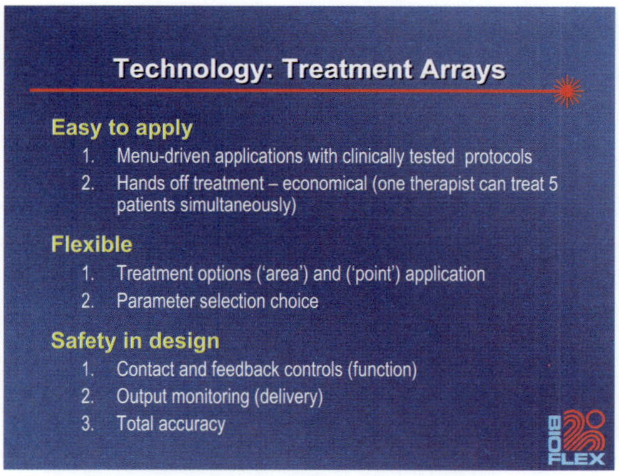

18.

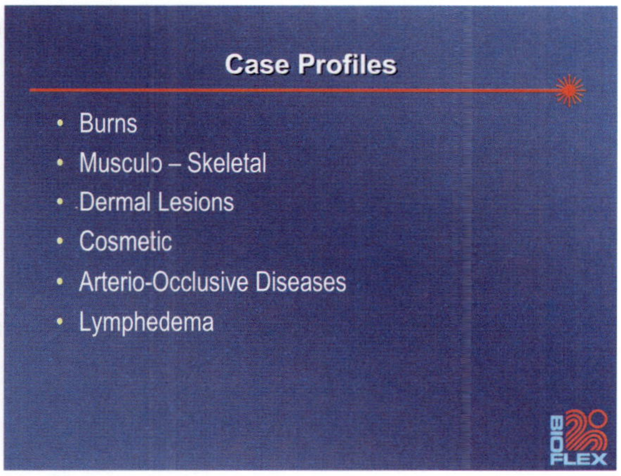

19.

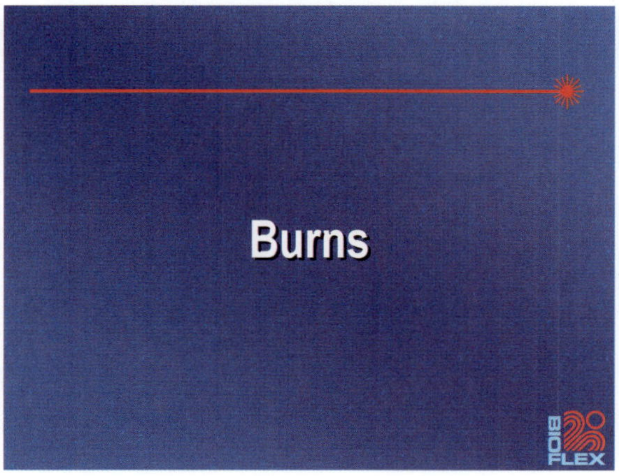

20.

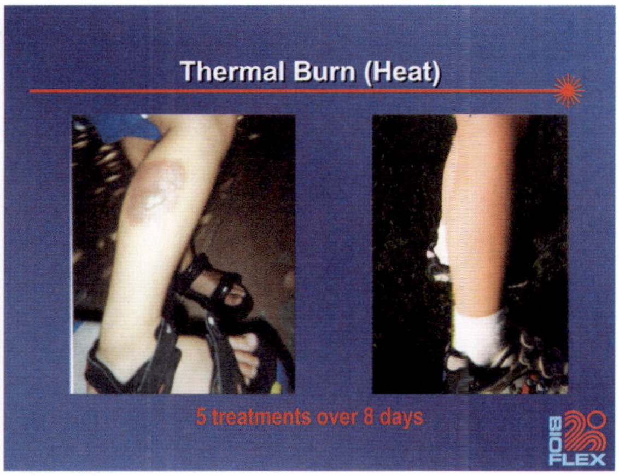

21.

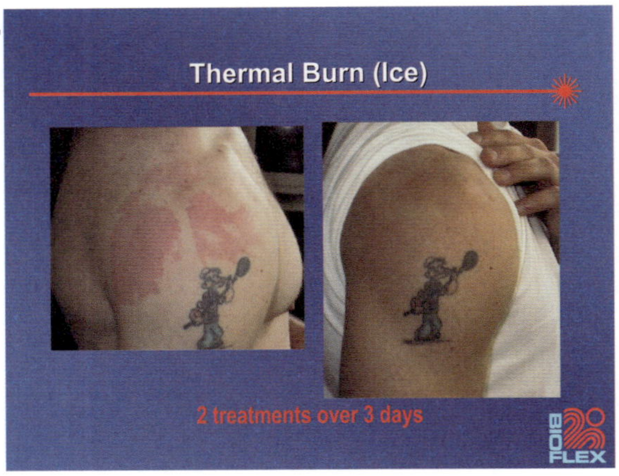

22.

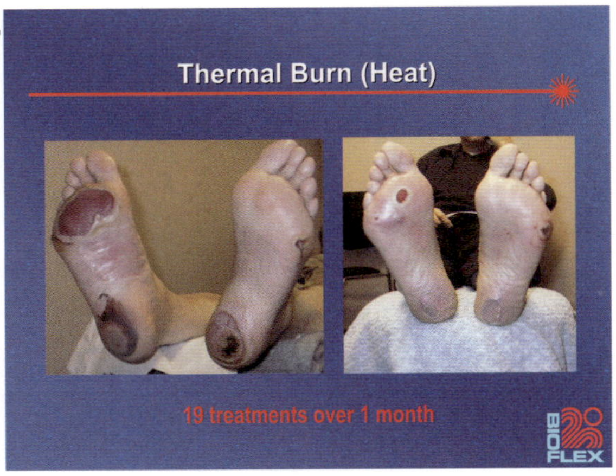

23.

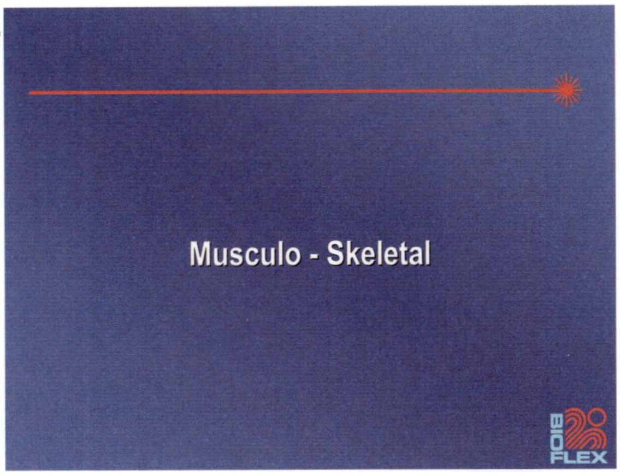

24.

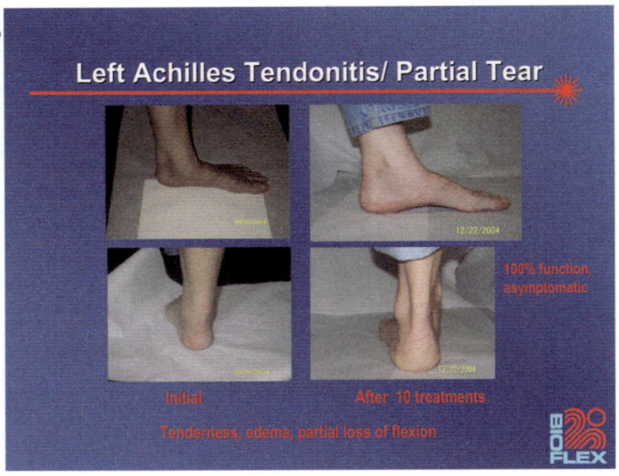

25.

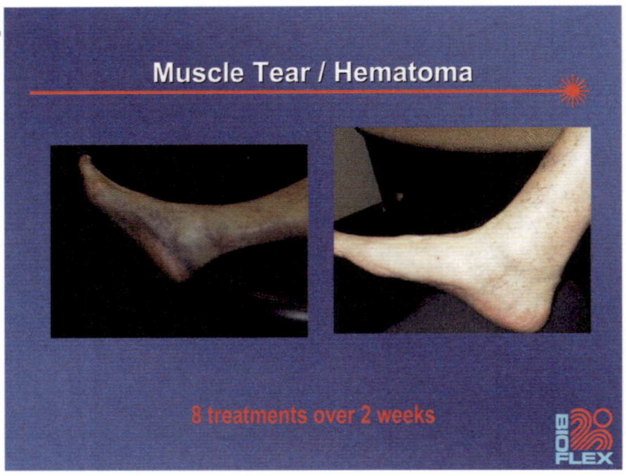

26.

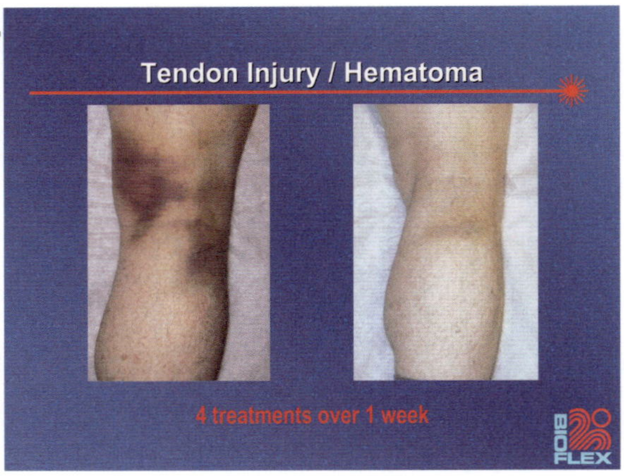

27.

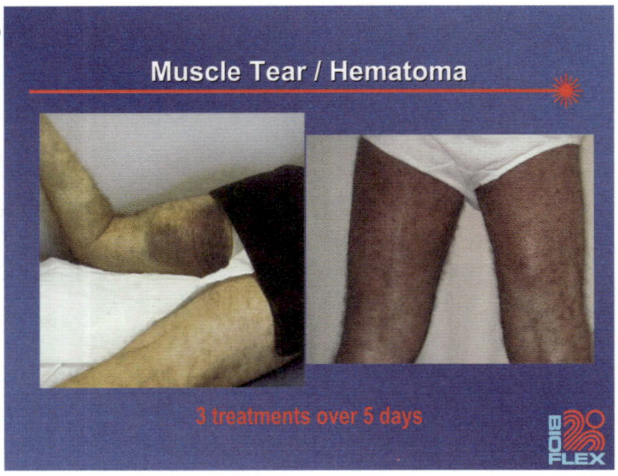

28.

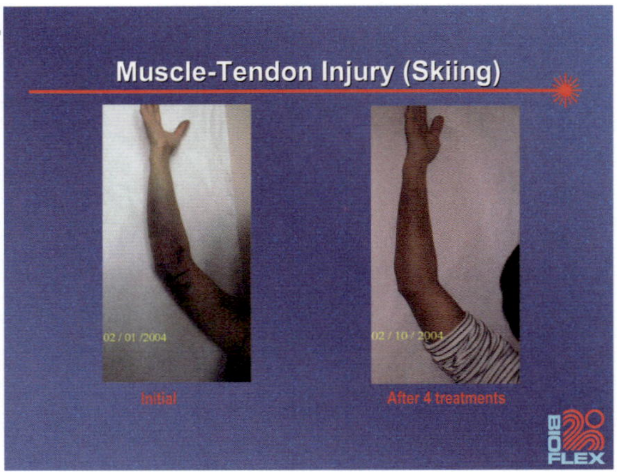

29.

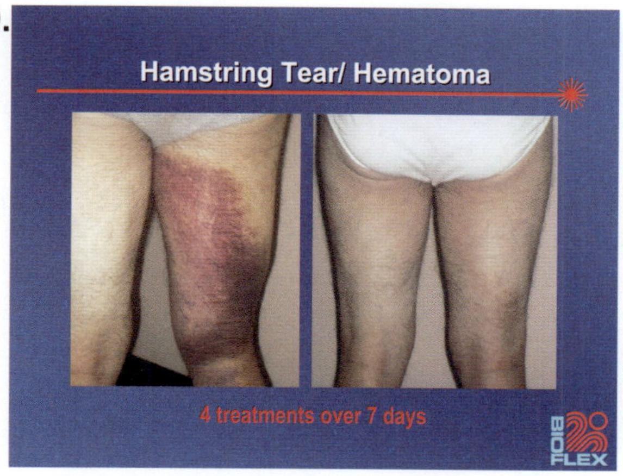

30.

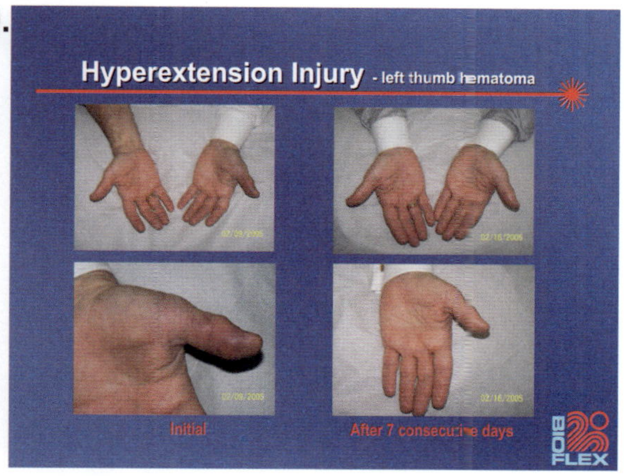

31.

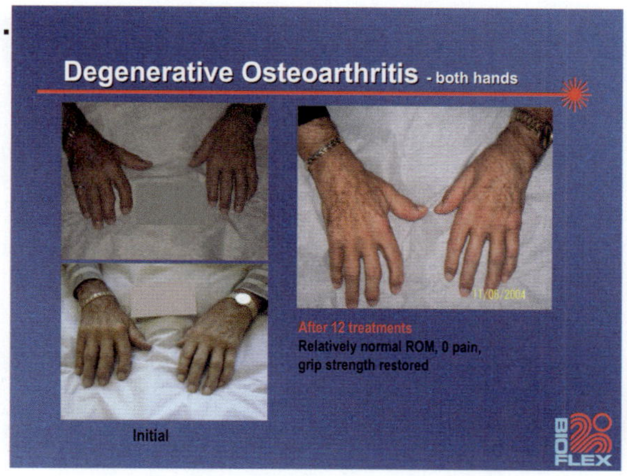

32.

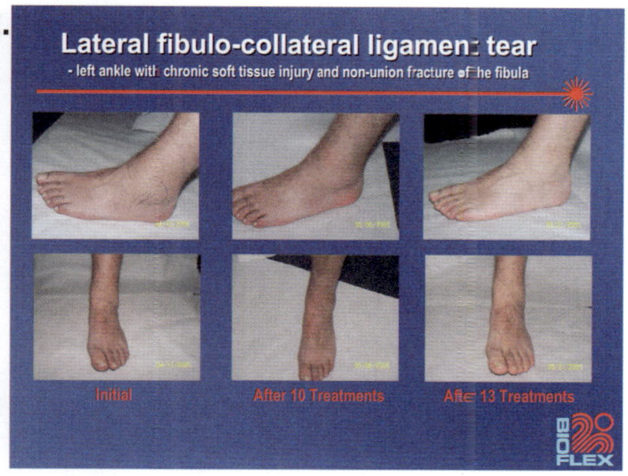

33.

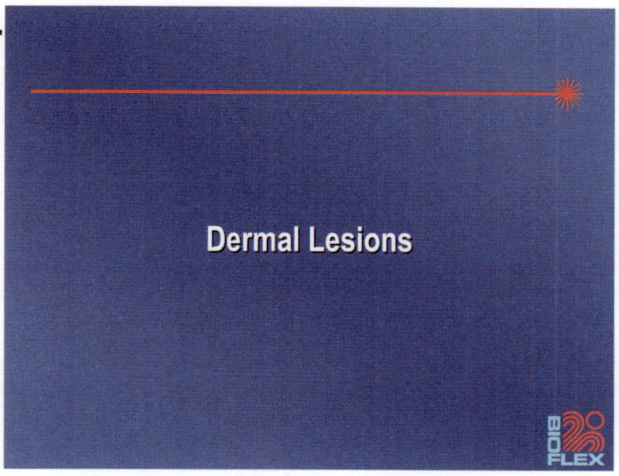

34.

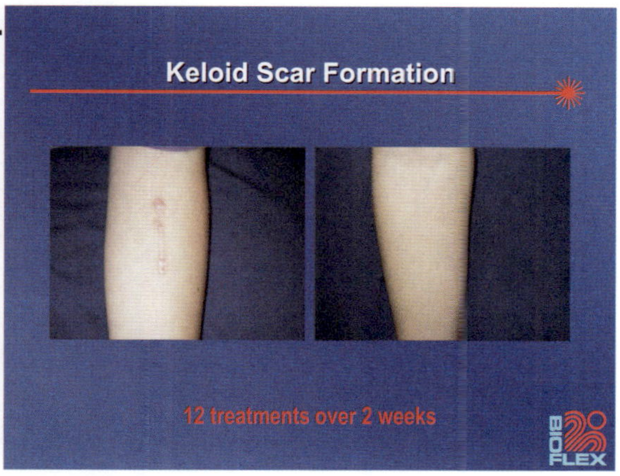

35.

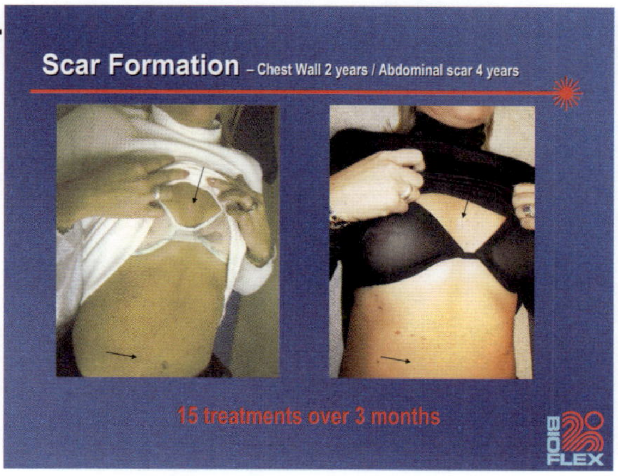

36.

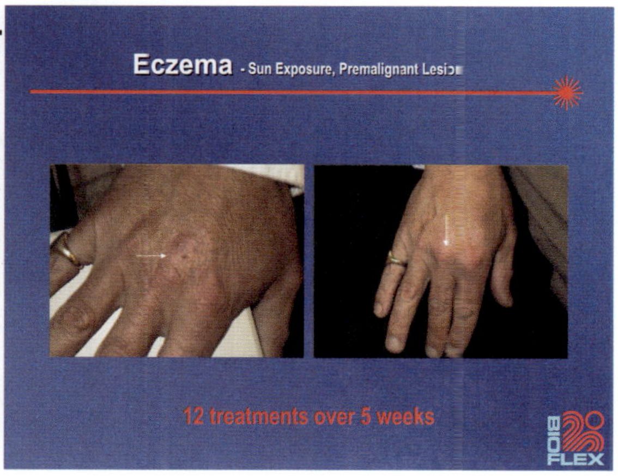

37.

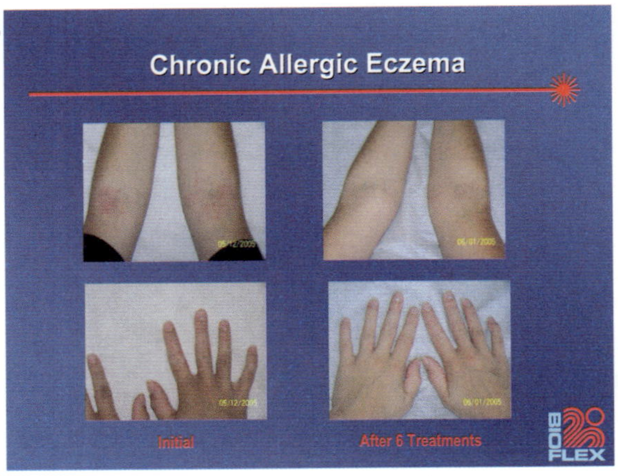

38.

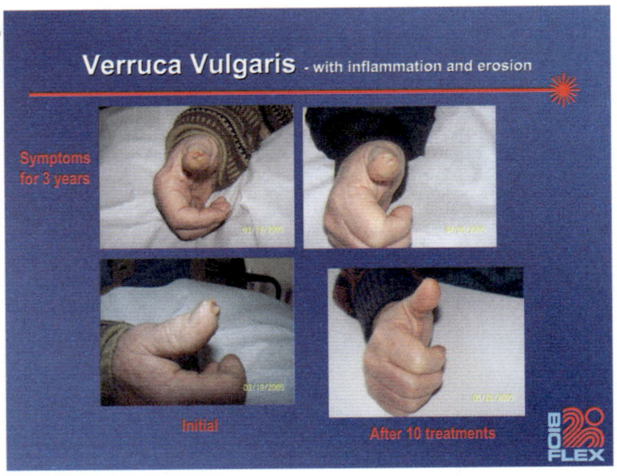

39.

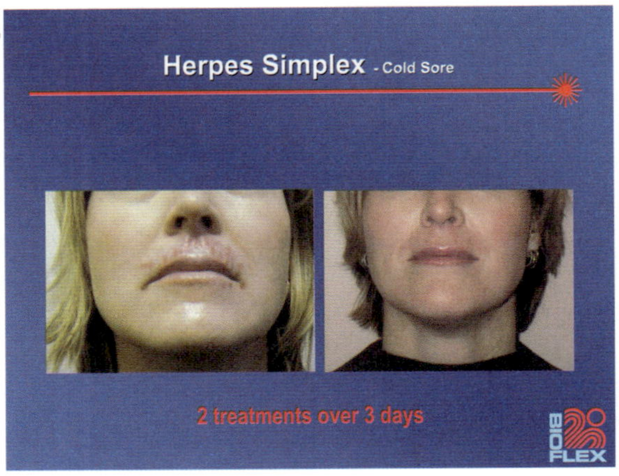

40.

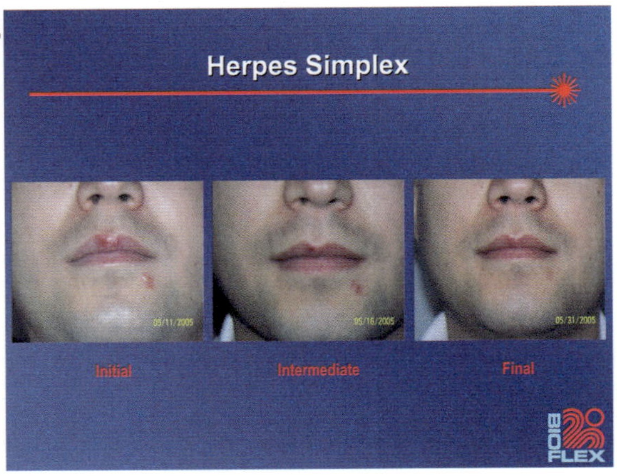

41.

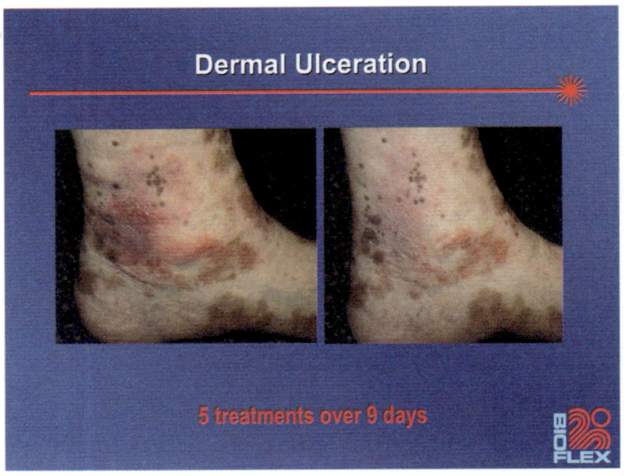

42.

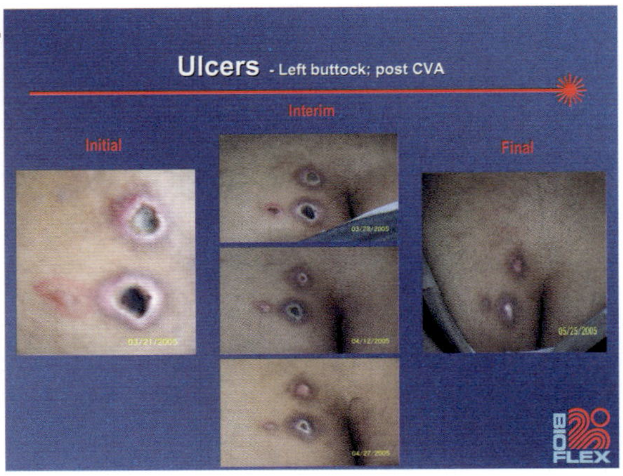

43.

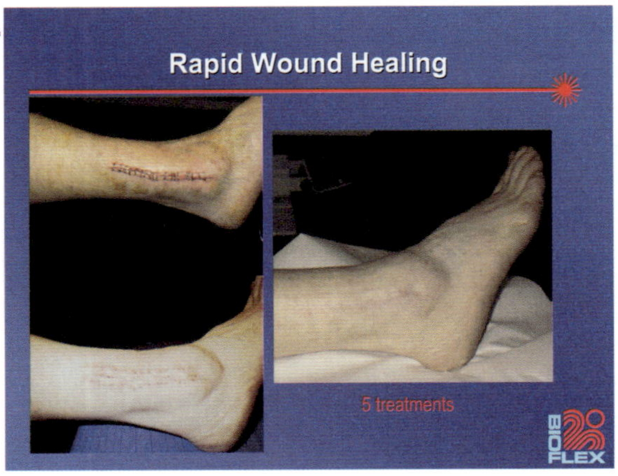

44.

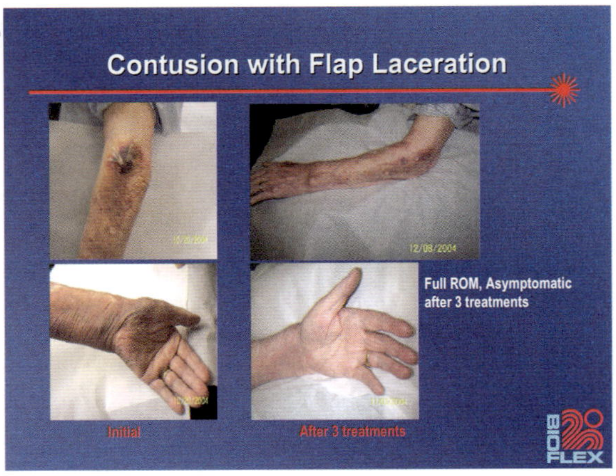

45.

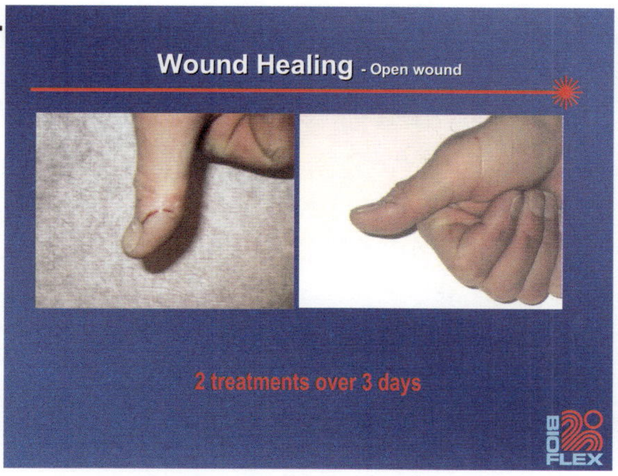

46.

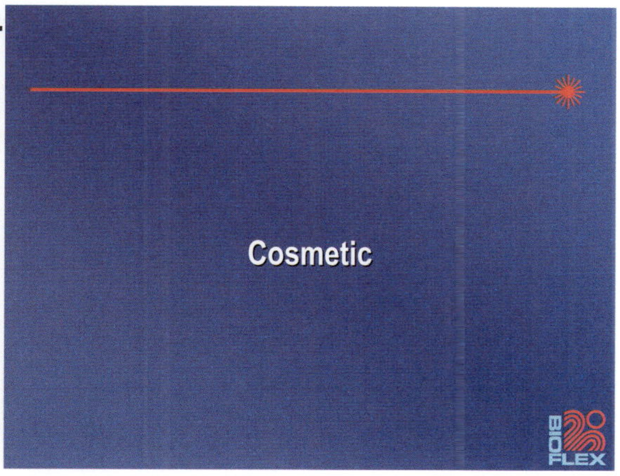

47.

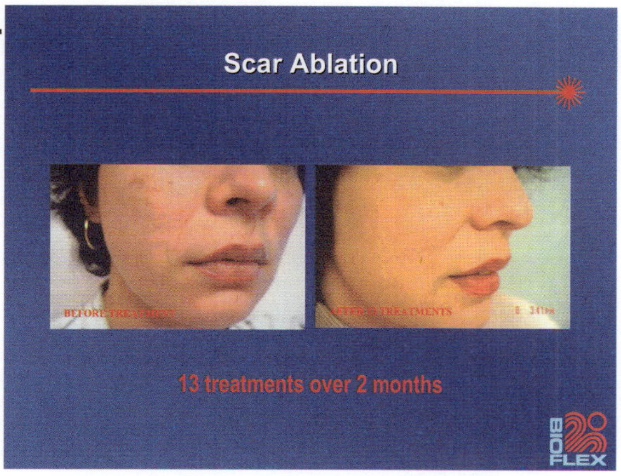

48.

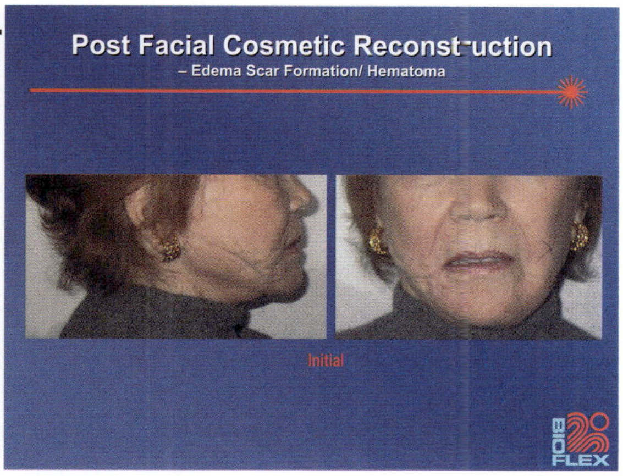

49.

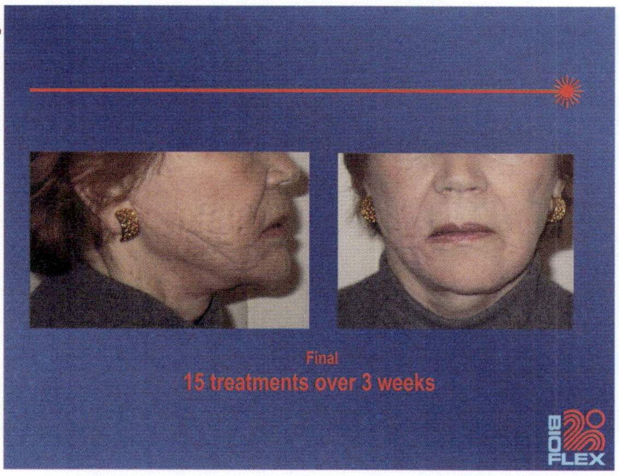

50.

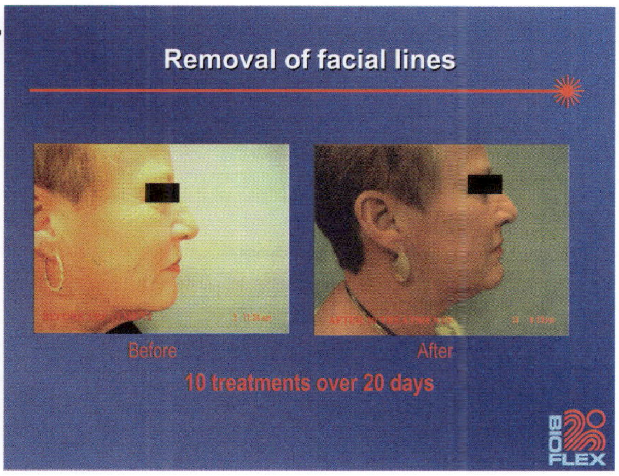

51.

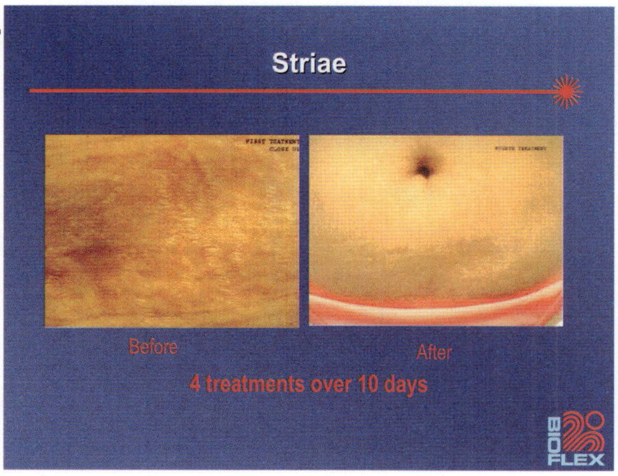

52.

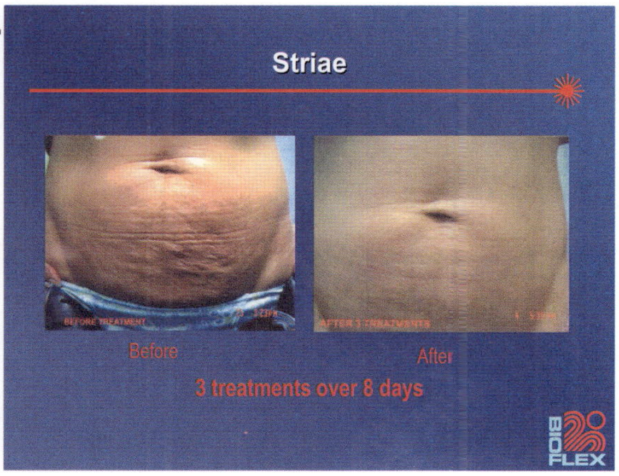

53.

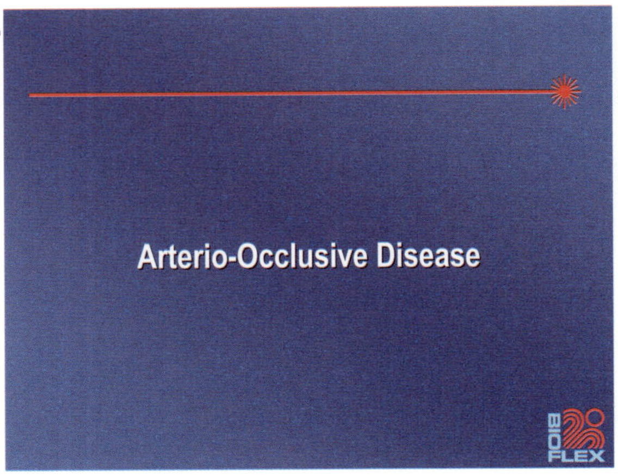

54.

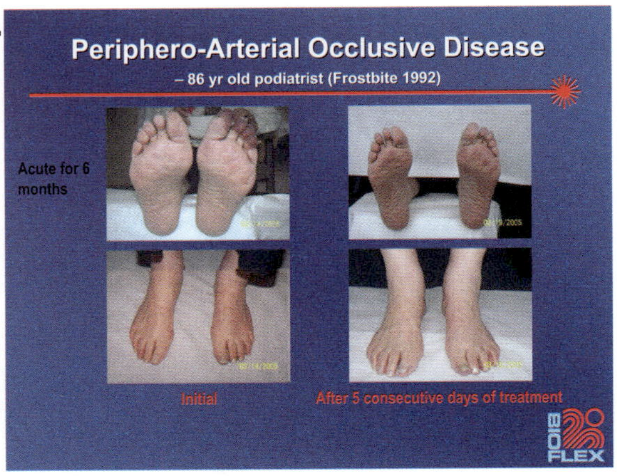

55.

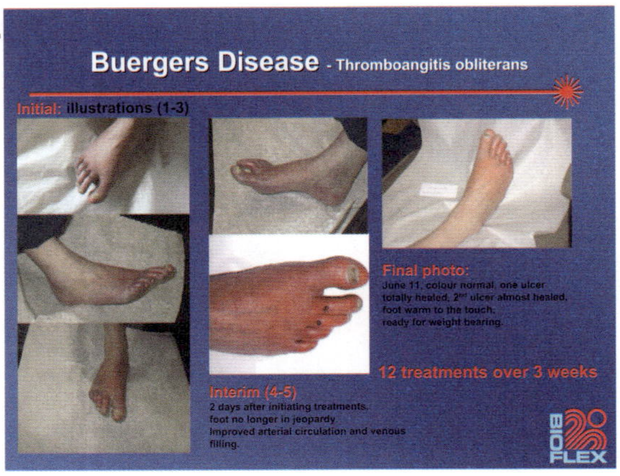

56.

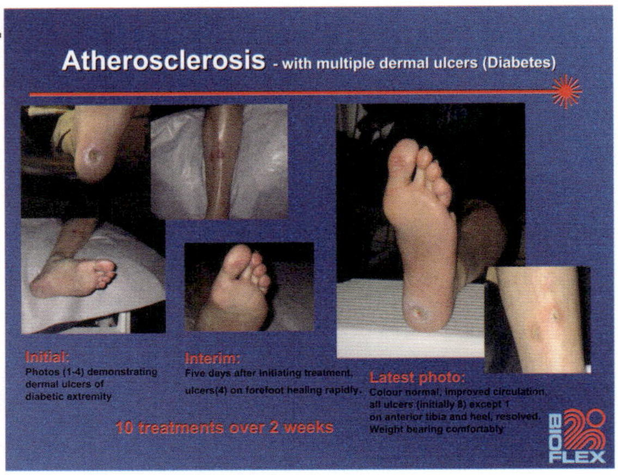

57.

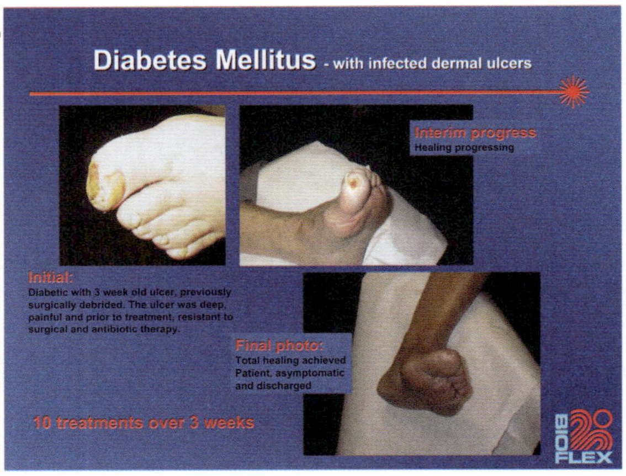

58.

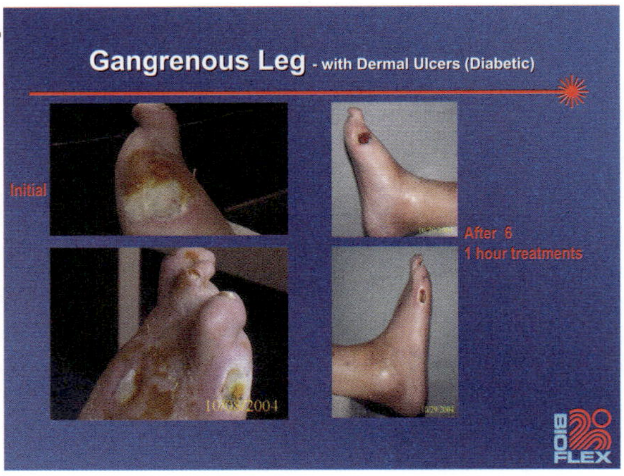

59.

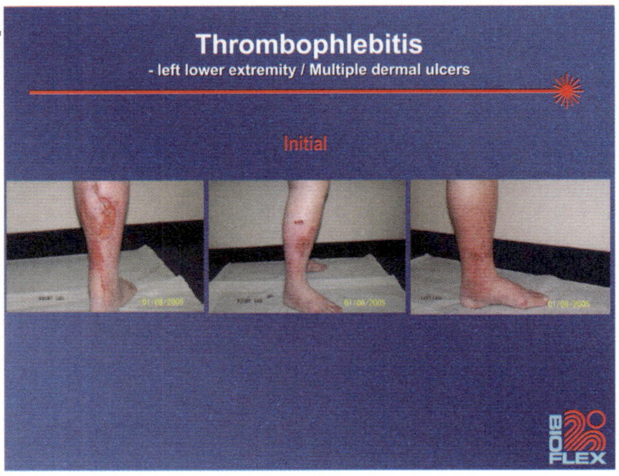

60.

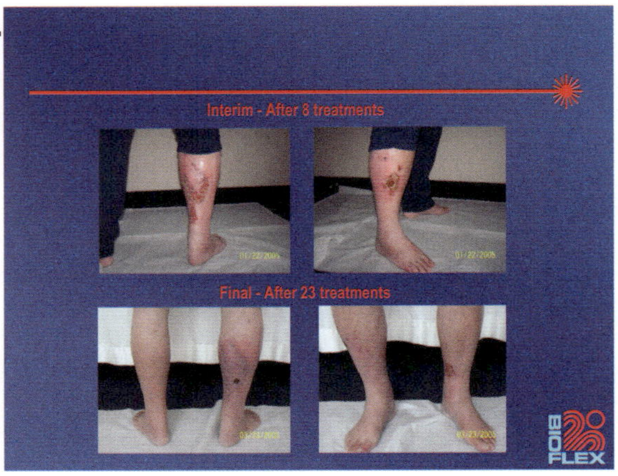

61.

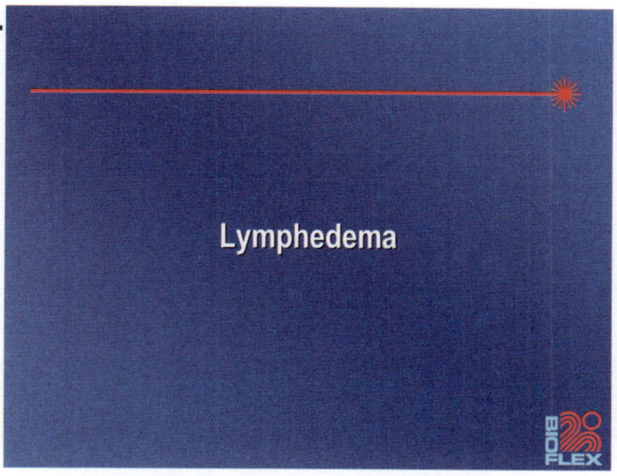

62.

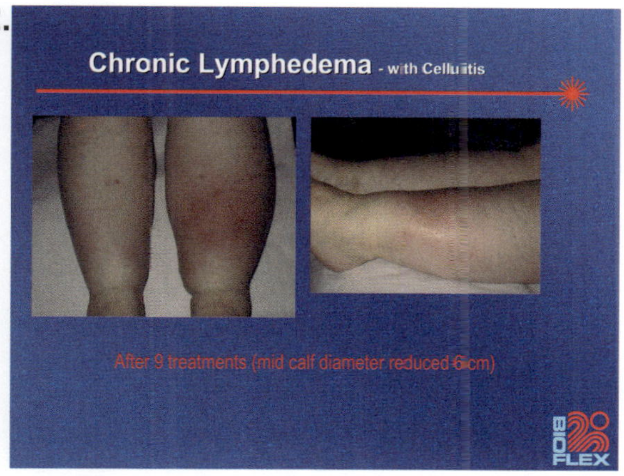

63.

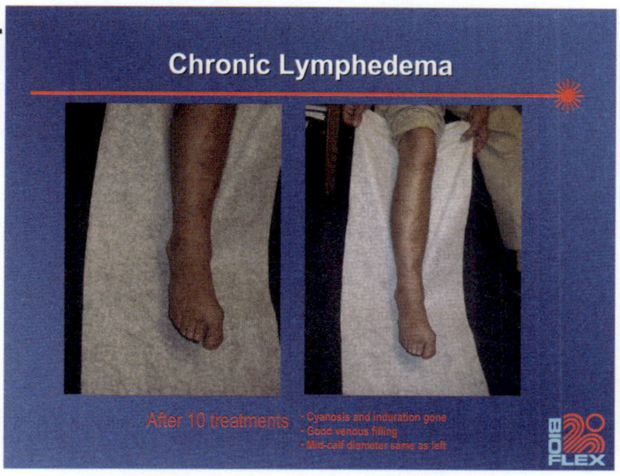

64.

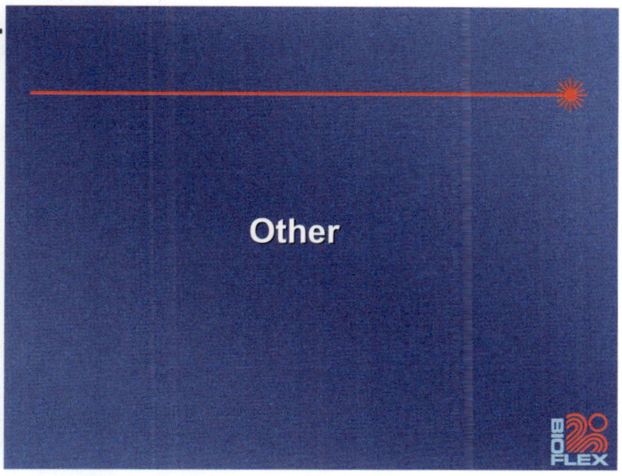

65.

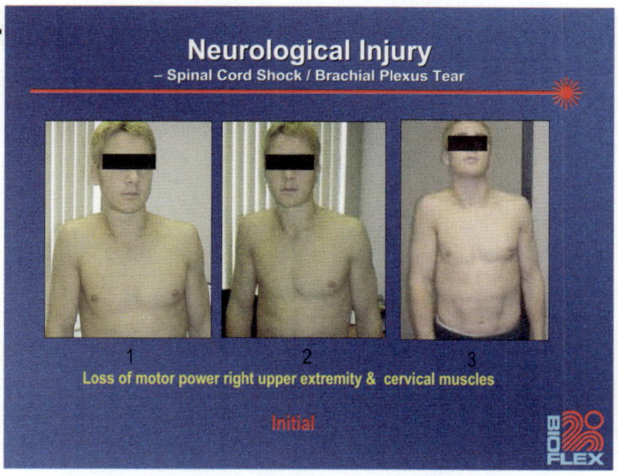

66.

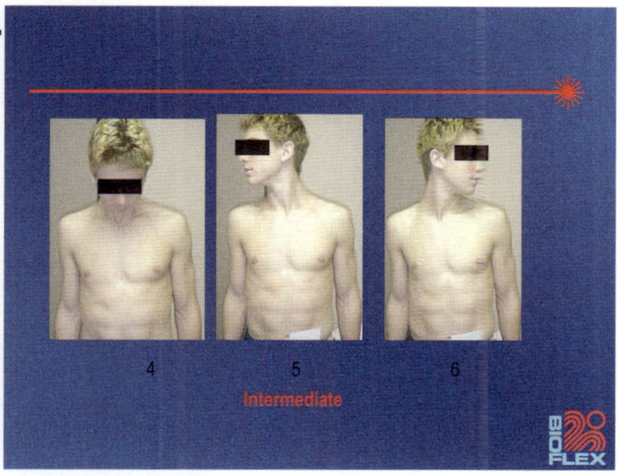

67.

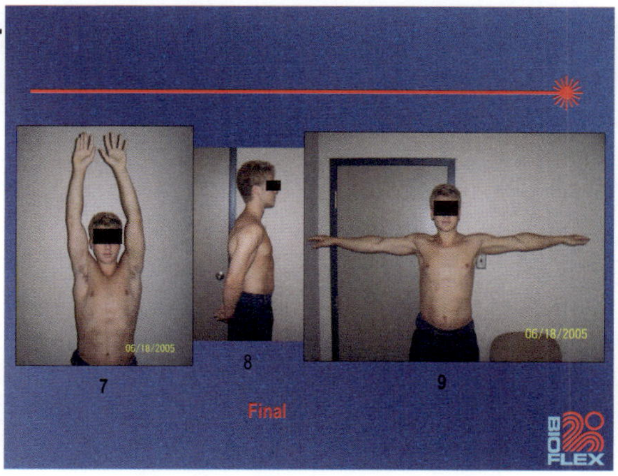

68.

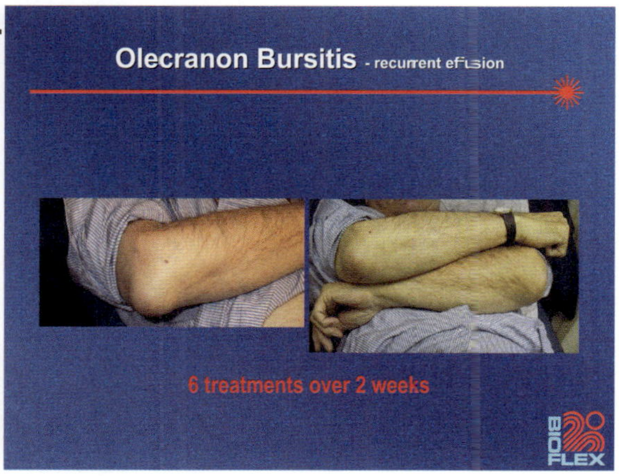

69.

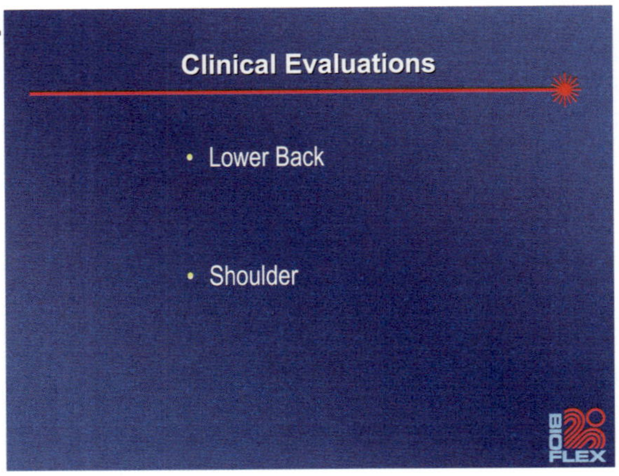

70.

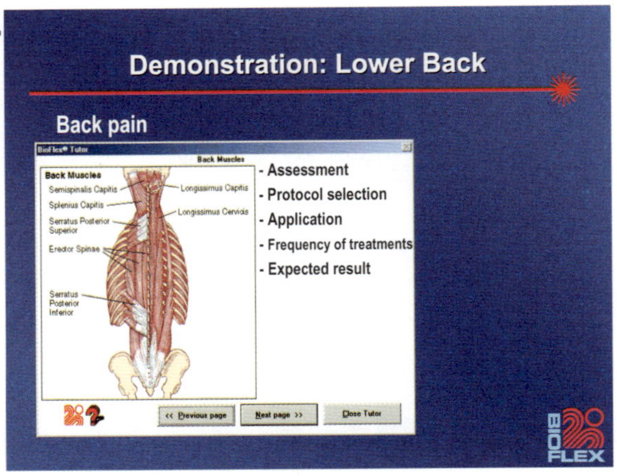

71.

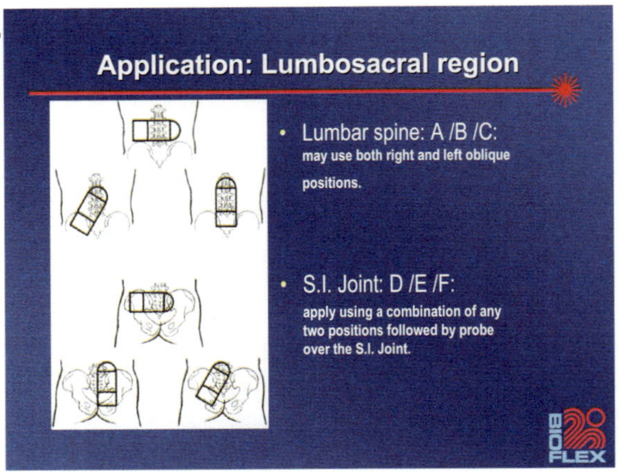

72.

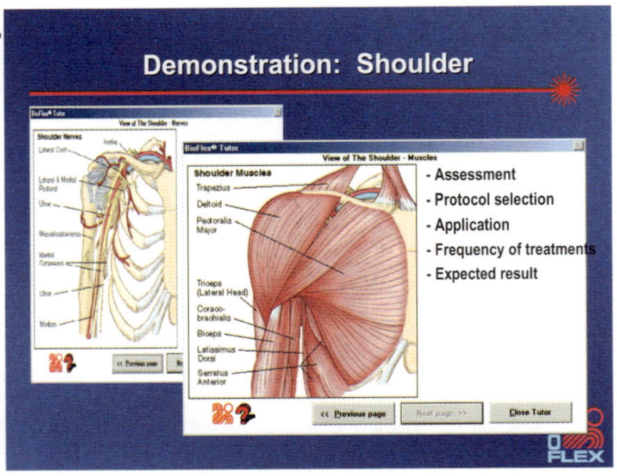

73.

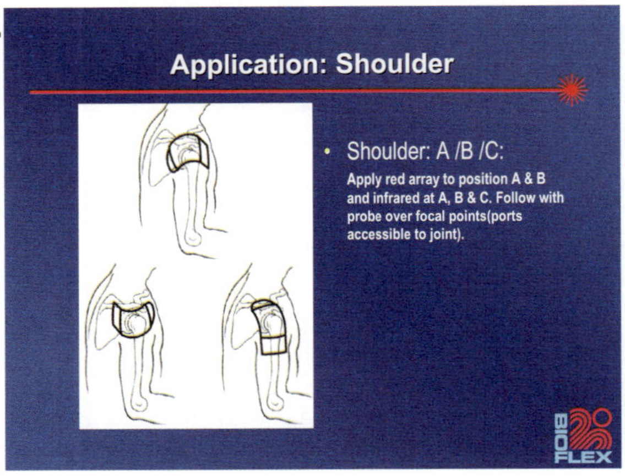

74.

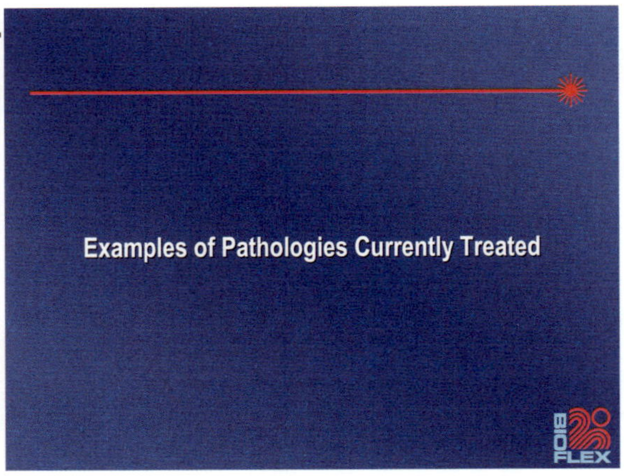

75.

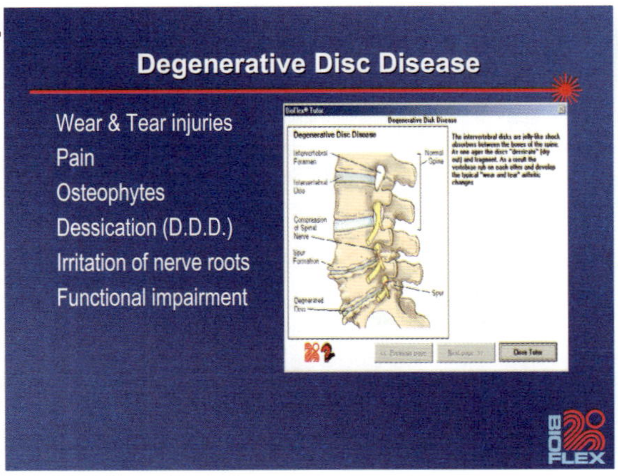

76.

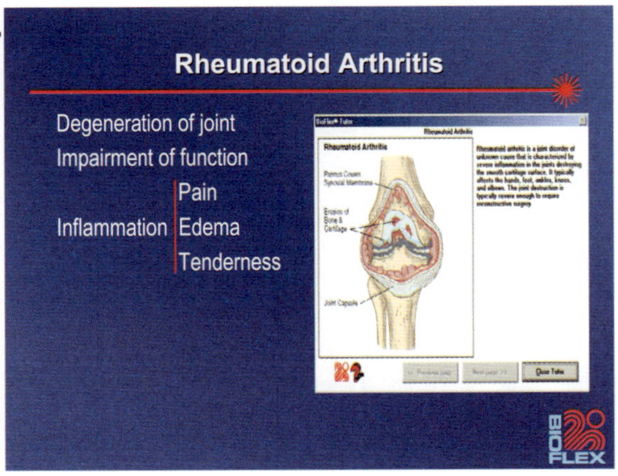

77.

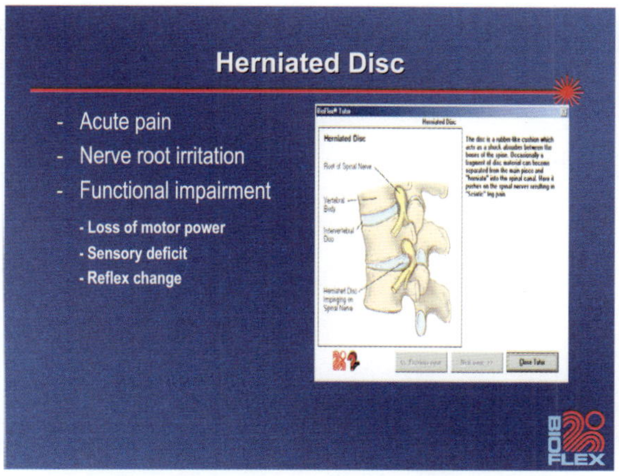

78.

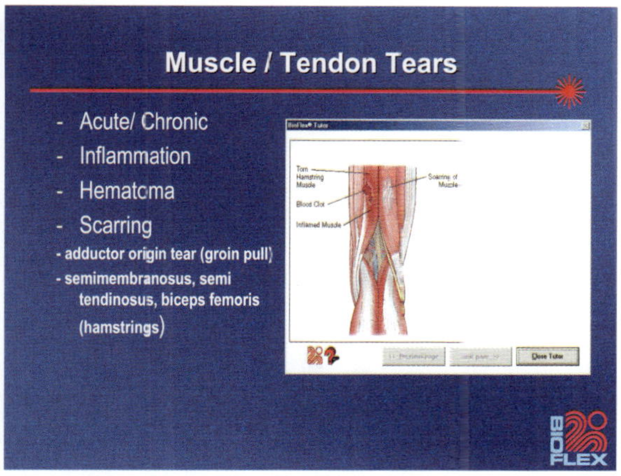

79.

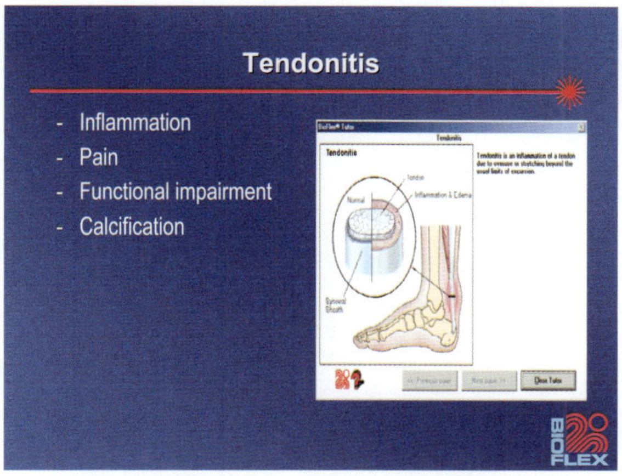

80.

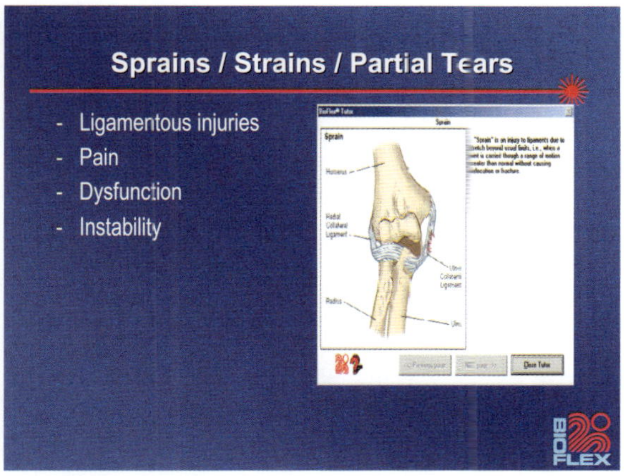

81.

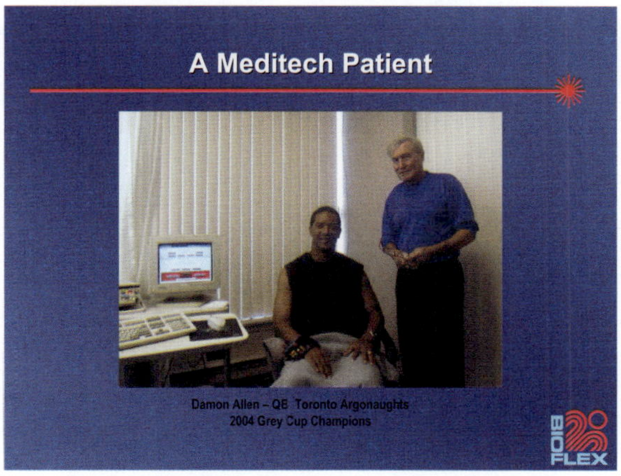

82.

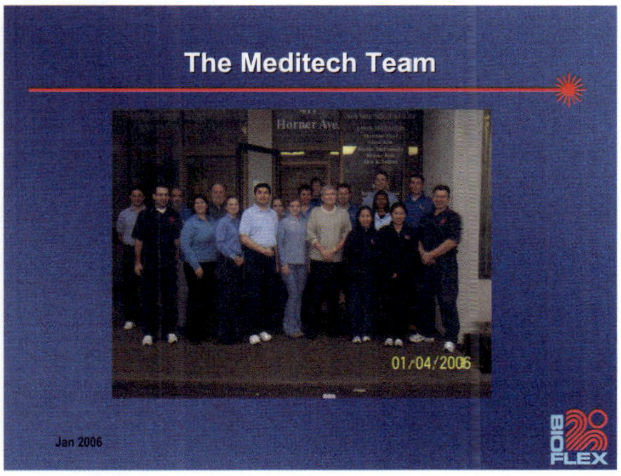

83.

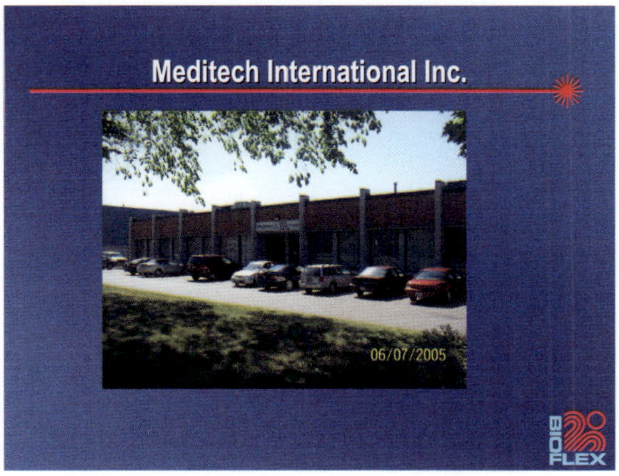

84.

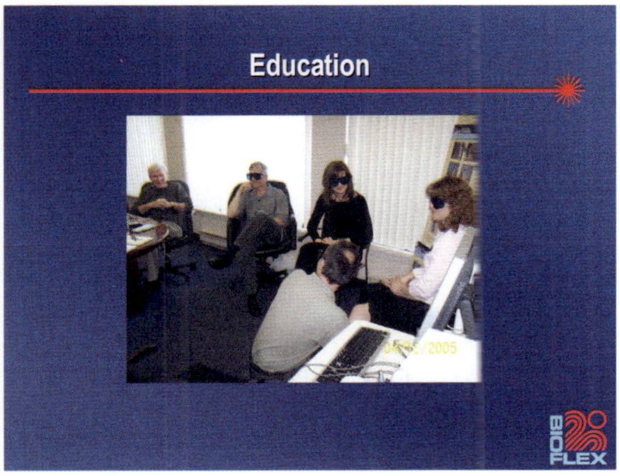

V Bibliography

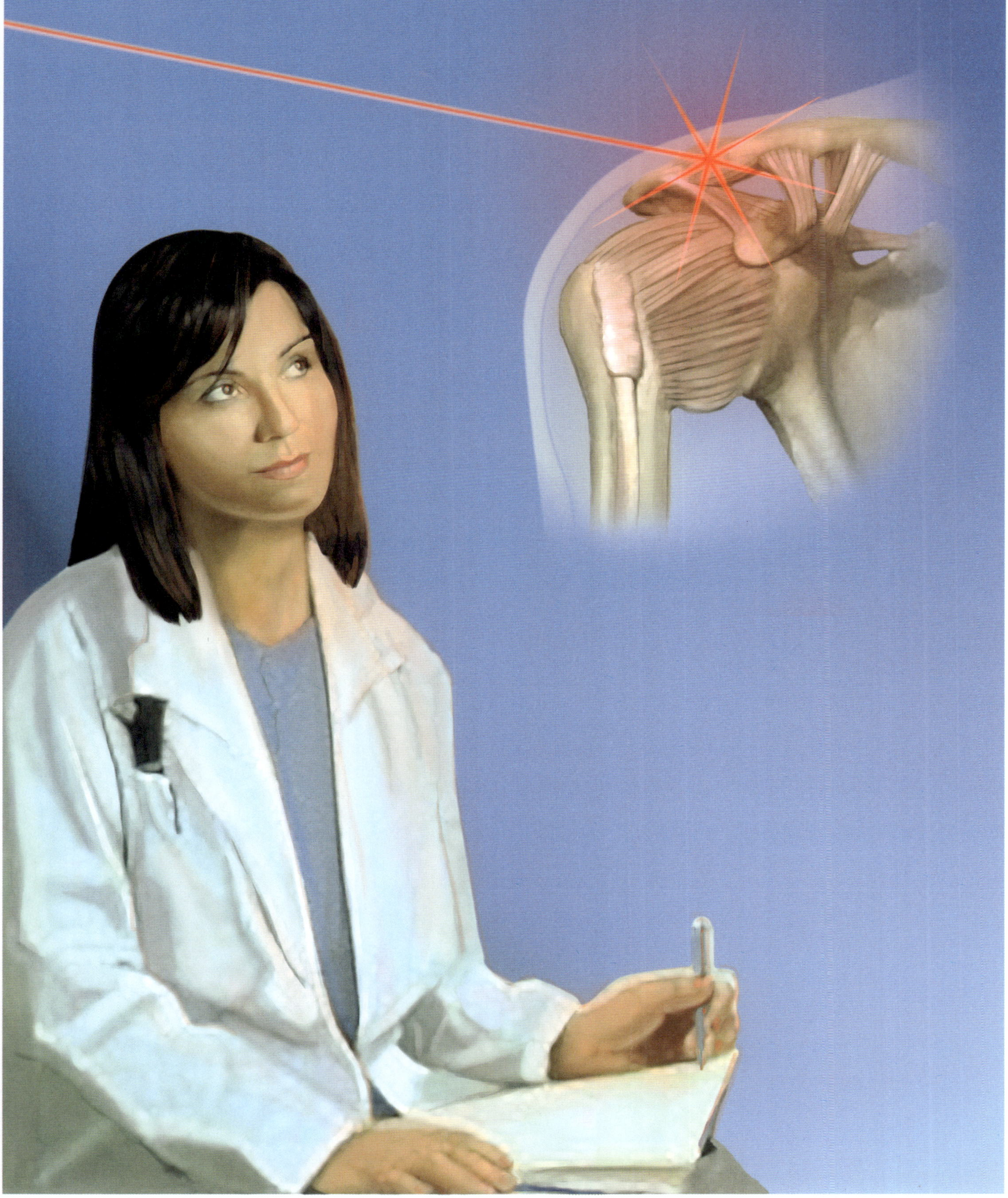

List of References

1. **Agaiby A, Ghali L, Dyson M** Laser modulation of T-lymphocyte proliferation in vitro. *Laser Therapy.* 1998 10:153-158.
2. **Brosseau L, Welch V, Wells G, Tugwell P, de Bie R, Gam A, Harman K, Shea B, Morin M,** Low Level Laser Therapy for osteoarthritis and rheumatoid arthritis: a meta analysis. *J. Rheumattol* 2000 Aug; 27(8):1961-9.
3. **Carati CJ, Anderson SN, Gannon BJ, Piller NB**. Treatment of postmastectomy lymphedema with low-level laser therapy: a double blind, placebo-controlled trial. *Cancer.* 2003 Sept 15;98(6);1114-22.
4. **Dyson M**, Evidence Based Use of Light and other forms of Phototherapy for Tissue Repair., Dept of Physical Therapy and Rehabilitation Sciences, Kansas Medical Center, Kansas, USA 2003
5. **Dyson M, Agaiby A, Ghahi L.** Photobiomodulation of human T-lymphocyte proliferation in vitro. *Lasers Med Sci.* 2002 17(4):A22
6. **El Sayed S O, Dyson M,** Effect of Laser Pulse Repetition Rate and Pulse Duration on Mast Cell Number and Degranulation. *Lasers Surg Med* 1996; 19(4):433-7.
7. **Enwemeka C. et al.**, Biochemistry and Biomechanics of Healing Tendon: Part I. Effects of Combined Laser Therapy and Exercise. *Medicine and Science in Sports and Exercise.* Vol. 12, (2)., pp 794-799, 1997
8. **Ernst E, Fialka V,** Low Dose Laser Therapy: Critical Analysis of Clinical Effect. *Schweiz Med Wochenschr.* 1993 May 8; 123(18):949-54. Review
9. **Feinstein A, MS, MD**, Sterling Professor of Medicine and Epidemiology, Yale University School of Medicine. 'Translating Evidence into Practice 1998, Conference Summary. Agency for Health Care Policy and Research, Rockville, MD. http://www.ahrq.gov/clinic/trip1998/
10. **Gupta AK et al.** The use of low energy photon therapy (LEPT) in venous leg ulcers: a double blind, placebo-controlled study. *Am Soc Derm Surg* 1998 24:1383-1386
11. **Guyton, A.C. and Hall, J.E.**: Textbook of Medical Physiology.10th Edition, Philadelphia: W.B. Saunders Company, 2000.
12. **Hillsdon M, Thorogood M**, A Systemic Review of Physical Activity Promotion Strategies. *Br J Sports Med* 1996 Jun; 30(2): 84-9.
13. **Iijima K, Shimoyama N, Shimoyama M, Mizuguchi T.** Evaluation of analgesic effect of low-power He:Ne laser on postherpetic neuralgia using VAS and modified McGill pain questionnaire. *J Clin Laser Med Surg.* 1991 Apr;9(2);121-6.
14. **Kahn F**., Wound Healing, Case Profiles. 2005, Meditech International Inc.
15. **Kahn F.**, The Role of Low Intensity Laser Therapy in the maintenance of Optimal Health. A Review of 576 Consecutive Patient Discharges at the Meditech Clinic. Clinical Report. 2003, Meditech International Inc.
16. **Kahn F**, Low Intensity Laser Therapy in the Treatment of Periphero-Arterial Occlusive Disease., Clinical Study. 2004, Meditech International Inc.
17. **Kahn F,** Low Intensity Laser Therapy in the Treatment of Juvenile Rheumatoid Arthritis. A Case Study. 2000, Meditech International Inc.
18. **Kahn F, Graham M,** Low Intensity Laser Therapy in Clinical Practice, Clinical Study. 2000, Meditech International Inc.

19. **Kahn F, Stott M, Perrin LC,** The Relevance of Laser Therapy in Current Clinical Practice. Clinical Report 2002. Meditech International Inc.

20. **Kaput J, Rodriguez RL,** Nutritional Genomics: The Next Frontier in the Post genomic Era. *Physiol Genomics* 2004 Jan 15; 16(2): 166-77.

21. **Karu T.** Molecular mechanism of the therapeutic effect of low-intensity laser irradiation. *Lasers in the life Sciences*, 1988: 2:53-74.

22. **Karu T,**. Personal communications

23. **Karu T,** The Science of Low Power Laser Therapy, Gordon and Breach. *Science Publishers* 1997.

24. **Ohshiro T, Calderhead RG**, Development of Low Reactive-Level Laser Therapy and its Present Status, *J Clin Laser Med Surg*., Aug, 9(4); 267-75, 1991

25. **Piller NB, Thelander A.,** Treatment of Chronic Postmastectomy Lymphedema with Low Level Laser Therapy: a 2.5 year follow-up Study. *Lymphology* 31(2):74-86, 1998

26. **Rochkind S, Nissan M, Alon M et al.,** Effects of Laser Irradiation on the Spinal Cord for the Regeneration of Crushed Peripheral Nerve in Rats., *Lasers in Surgery and Medicine* 2001, 28(3):216-219.

27. **Rochkind S. et al.**, Double-Blind Randomized Study Using Neurotube and Laser Therapy in the Treatment of Complete Sciatic Nerve Injury in Rats. Proc. 2nd Congress World Assoc., for Laser Therapy. Kansas City, 1998.

28. **Rosch PJ**, Reminiscences of Hans Selye and the birth of "Stress". *Int J Emerg Ment Health* 1999 Winter; 1(1):59-66.

29. **Schindl A, Neumann R,** Low Intensity Laser Therapy is an Effective Treatment for Recurrent Herpes Simplex Infection. Results from a Randomized Double-Blind Placebo-Controlled Study.*The Journal of Investigative Dermatology*. Vol. 113, No. 2, August 1999.

30. **Schindl A, Schindl M**, Pernerstorfer-Schon H, Schindl L, Low Intensity Laser Therapy: A Review. *J Investig Med* 2000 Sept; 48(5):312-26. Review

31. **Sherry S**, Frustrations with Clinical Trials. *Eur J Clin Pharmacol.* 1980 Feb;17(2):79-80.

32. **Simunovic Z, Trobonjaca T, Trobonjaca Z**, Treatment of Medical and Lateral Epicondylitis – Tennis and Golfer's Elbow – with Low Level Laser Therapy: a Multicenter Double Blind, placebo-controlled Clinical Study on 324 Patients. Laser Centre Locarno, Switzerland. tzlatko@mamed.medri.hr , *J Clin Laser Med Surg* 1998 Jun; 16(3): 145-51

33. **Smyth J A**, Determining Optimal Therapy-Randomized Trials in Individual Patients. *N Engl J Med.* 1986 Sept 18;315(12):767-8.

34. **Sommer SJ**, Mind-Body Medicine and Holistic Approaches. The Scientific Evidence. *Aust Fam Physician* 1996 Aug; 25(8): 1233-7, 1240-1, 1244.

35. **Tuner J, Hode L,** It's All in the Parameters: A Critical Analysis of Some Well-known Negative Studies on Low Level Laser Therapy. *J Clin Laser Med Surg.* 1998 Oct; 16(5):245-8. Review

36. **Turner, J. and L. Hode**. Laser therapy clinical background and scientific practice, 13.3, Prima Books AB, Grängesberg, 2002.

37. **Van Kampen K**, Triumph of the Pill. A Story of Health, Wealth and Stealth. *National Post, Business.*, September 2002.

38. **Vladimirov YA, Osipov AN, Klebanov GI**, Photobiological Principles of Therapeutic Applications of Laser Radiation. *Biochemistry (Moscow)*, Vol 69, No 1, 2004, pp. 81-90.

39. **Walker J**, Relief from Chronic Pain by Low Power Laser Therapy, Neuroscience Letters, 43(1983) 339-344

40. **Wente M**, Why Health Care will Never Be Reformed. *Globe and Mail,* Counterpoint, October 2002.

41. **Yaksich I, Tan LC, Previn V.** Low energy laser therapy for treatment of post-herpetic neuralgia. *Ann Acad Med Singapore.* 1993 May;22(3 Suppl);441-2.

42. **Zlatko S**, Low Level Laser Therapy with Trigger Points Technique: A study on 243 Patients. FMH Journal of Clin. *Laser Medicine & Surgery*, (1996) V 14, No. 4, pp. 163-167.

List of Tables

List of Figures

Glossary of Terms

Eye Shield: Medical Grade Eye Shields that protect the eyes totally(100% block) from any radiation. Eye shields are used by the patient during Low Intensity Laser Treatment on the face.

Generic Prescription: A treatment protocol that is specific for the type of pathology but not specific for the location on the body to be treated.

Good Contact: Low Intensity Laser Therapy systems must provide good physical contact between the treatment head (diodes) and the surface of the area being treated, in order to ensure efficient and reliable delivery of light energy to the target tissue. The BioFlex Professional System is designed for this type of contact and has feedback systems that ensure it takes place.

LILT: LILT is an acronym for Low Intensity Laser Therapy. It is synonymous with LLLT, the acronym for Low Level Laser Therapy. Unlike the high intensity medical lasers used to thermally cut and coagulate tissues, LILT involves the use of medical lasers that operate at intensities too low to damage living tissues. Their action is photobiomodulation; they can stimulate damaged tissue components(Kahn F, 1999, Agaihy et al 1998; Dyson, Agaihy & Ghali 2002).

Prescription: A treatment protocol that is the embodiment of many successful clinical applications of specific parameters (Frequency(Hz), Duty Cycle(%), Wave Form(Square/ Sine/ Triangle), Duration(sec.), Mode of Operation (Modulated/ Continuous/ Pulsed) wave, Wave Length(nm), Treatment Head(Superluminous Array, Laser Probe), Energy Density(j/cm2), and Power Density(Watts/cm2). Prescriptions are presented in three(3) stages.

Safety Glasses: A wave length specific filter covering the eyes for protection against laser beams that may be prevalent in a treatment area. Safety Glasses must be worn by the therapist as well as the patient being treated.

Safety Policy for Application of Low Intensity Laser Therapy: Safe application of LILT is accomplished if a) Both patient and therapist are protected with wavelength specific eye glasses, from the laser source in use, b) The treatment area is secure from the surroundings with protection from accidental release of laser light, and c) The laser device in use is operating correctly.

Sandwich Approach: The application of a Treatment Array around an anatomical part so that the light beam enters the anatomical part (such as a wrist) from more than one(1) side, surrounding the area and concentrating the light.

Stage I, II & III: Stages I, II & III are considered entry points for a specific treatment. All patients are different. The treatment protocol selected should satisfy the requirements for treating the specific pathology considering the unique circumstances of the individual patient. Assessment and protocol selection are skills that take practice, experience and keen medical knowledge to apply.

Treatment Array: A flexible treatment head that provides a healing light source in a flexible device to enable efficient and complete delivery of light to any anatomical configuration.

Social Commentary #1

The Canadian Heath Care System

Nothing seems to capture the attention of Canadians more than Medicare. Since its inception in Saskatchewan, the concept of collectively sharing the cost of illness and injury has become a defining character of what it means to be Canadian. From coast to coast, healthcare apparently is both a public responsibility and a “free” service. Decreed by the Canada Health Act, Canadians believe themselves universally entitled to comprehensive, accessible, publicly administered healthcare that is portable. The principles of the Canada Health Act are unfortunately unrealistic.

Two fundamentally economic principles underlie the financial problems of Medicare. The demand for any free good goods is infinite, notwithstanding the fact that few people choose to be ill. Second, no goods or services are free; someone must pay for the provisions thereof.

The Problems Relating To The Act:

1. Public expectations of what Medicare is - the desire for all health needs to be covered.
2. High and continuing escalation of costs for the foreseeable future due to advancing technologies.
3. An expanding aging population that will place ongoing demands on the current system for years to come.
4. Rationing of services is problematic as it is contrived by insufficient funds. It deprives those in true need from accessing services that are required and frequently supposes that one person’s suffering is more worthy of consideration than anothers.
5. The Canada Act is an immoral act in that it has forced upon even those who would otherwise afford to relieve their own suffering and the right of the individual to pursue a course of therapy that will relieve their symptoms expeditiously and in an acceptable manner.
6. The present system is inefficient as there is no alignment of goals and no pressures to force efficiency. Health institutions are virtually a monopoly within the system. Public confidence is being rapidly eroded by perpetual wrangling over who pays and the lack of clarity as to the long term commitment of governments which must be defined.

Possible Approaches to Saving Medicare:

1. To spend more money without making changes – the easy fix – for the short term till demand exceeds supply – again.
2. Establish a formula for funding Medicare and define clearly what it will and will not cover. Make an irrevocable commitment to a minimum level of funding and ensure that there is a good health system for all that need it and choose to use it. We cannot abandon those in true need who do not have sufficient means.
3. Create a genuine health service system and achieve within it greater cost

effectiveness by introducing competition and accountability even if it does not include "for profit" organizations. Nothing stirs the innovative mind more than competition where ones own existence may be at stake.

4. Increase choice and simultaneously reduce rationing by permitting those that choose to do so the opportunity to relieve their own suffering by paying directly for services they choose to consume. Support this by allowing the sale of health insurance. There is no shortage of physical beds in the hospital or surgeons willing to perform surgery – there is a shortage of funds to allow them to work as they should.

Discussion:

Whereas the system in principle encompasses the appropriate values, it has become increasingly flawed with regard to implementation and operation. The reasons for this are numerous. There is a diminishing focus on what the system should attempt to achieve, i.e. good patient care delivered in appropriate fashion with regard to timeliness and expedience.

There is an overwhelming demand and focus on documentation at the federal, provincial and regional level. The system should be streamlined under one body that understands healthcare, i.e. administration by properly qualified professionals rather than a bureaucracy that lacks understanding.

The numerous commissions, committees and consultants employed by various levels of government in the final analysis add nothing to the equation. These are costly, time consuming and focused on political and other considerations, rather than the delivery of quality healthcare to Canadian citizens.

The status of professionals continues to erode with increasing audits, restrictive covenants and harassment on all levels from the administrative sector, insurance companies and other bodies that have the right to regulate the medical profession. In fact they only serve to anger healthcare professionals to the degree where they lose focus and subconsciously punish the patient with regard to appropriate care. It is an extremely serious and negative factor as evidenced by high quality physicians still emigrating to the U.S. or physicians retiring from practice earlier than desirable.

The average Canadian has difficulty accessing the healthcare system unless it s a true "life and death" situation and sometimes even that may not be possible.

The press relentlessly preaches that the healthcare system here "is envied by the world". This is incorrect. Generally the average Canadian is required to undergo diagnostic studies and specialist consultation a period which takes between 3 months to a year. The time loss is unnecessary, causes much suffering and has significant economic impact. When serious illness occurs, diagnosis should follow and treatment be instituted within 24 hours or less. This could save vast amounts of wasted funds. One-third or more of all practice costs could be reduced by following this rather simple approach.

Affluent Canadians regardless of what the media states, can plug into the system quite easily through medical friends, hospital boards, etc. There is therefore a serious inequality on all levels and this is patently clear to the majority of participants within the delivery system.

The physician referral system is an abomination. Patients get bounced from one specialist to another and again there are immense gaps from the time the patient is seen by the family practitioner to the time a diagnosis is established. Therapeutic solutions are therefore unduly delayed. This causes increasing backups in the system to the point where it becomes unmanageable. Evidence of this is seen by the crowding in hospital emergency rooms, in practitioners and specialist offices where patients are generally met by nonresponsive, unsympathetic staff, including physicians. Growing waiting lists are the order of the day.

Increasingly, medicine today focuses on paperwork, administration and insurance company policies not to mention the patient chart which under the auspices of various regulatory bodies requires an increasing amount of unnecessary verbiage. No patient's health status was ever improved by excessive attention to paperwork or tests. The system in general leads to excessive investigations in the form of unnecessary tests and more importantly, excessive prescribing particularly for the elderly. Unquestionably this is another deleterious aspect of medical practice today. A sequence of consultants order multiple prescriptions, frequently with toxic and even fatal results.

Synopsis:

1. The administrative process should be streamlined with less focus on codes, accounting, paperwork and audits.
2. The system must return to a position of substance rather than style, i.e. address patient's health issues and institute therapy in a timely fashion.
3. Reduce the impact of the pharmaceutical industry. Many medications are useful and beneficial, however over 70% create more problems than they solve. Physicians are conditioned from the day they enter medical school to prescribe. This pressure must be reduced and more focus must be placed on education, prevention and alternative therapies.
4. The pharmaceutical industry's influence must be removed from medical schools, research centres and universities except as indicated on an appropriate basis.

In brief the current model of medical practice must undergo some radical revision with less emphasis on administration and more on patient care.

Social Commentary #2

Managed Health Care

Much as Celebrex and Vioxx were hailed as the panacea for arthritis, Managed Health Care was advertised as the proverbial savior of health care systems throughout the world a decade or so ago.

With the much-hyped takeover of medical practice by the corporate sector, the people believed that healthcare would be magically transformed. All problems would be solved, cost effectiveness would be the keynote and all patients would receive the ideal care that everyone desires and deserves. All that would be necessary was to sign up with a recommended provider, either under the corporate umbrella at no cost, or for the private citizen at minimal cost.

The corporate intelligentsia i.e. HMOs and insurance companies in alliance with and the approval of governments, (if the politicians in power thought it would bring in votes and increase their personal and election coffers,) were suddenly in concert. It was an assault that would bring the ultimate in healthcare to everyone i.e. accessibility, universality, affordability, freedom of choice, all bandied about in advertising slogans, like manna from heaven. No longer would the greedy doctors control healthcare but would become providers only, contracted by the new gate keepers. Just retribution for those who would prey on the misery of others for personal profit.

What has transpired? Over the past five years Celebrex, Vioxx and the other miracle drugs are literally and justifiably gone. Managed Health Care has proven to be nothing more than another "corporate profit grab" taking the majority of dollars out of the healthcare system for the personal gain of a few. Initially, lauded by Wall Street, Madison Avenue and a collection of major league law firms, the conventional corporate profiteers raped the system and created a multitude of billionaires and more than a few millionaires while taking patient care to new lows.

In the "prehistoric" fee-for-service system, physicians provided care directly to patients and were compensated by the client to the best of that individual's ability. It is safe to assume in that arrangement, 90% of healthcare dollars went towards patient care. Under the corporate and government umbrella 80% of healthcare dollars are "eaten up" by management and only 20% are available to pay the actual providers of care, an interesting statistic indeed.

To some extent doctors must shoulder a significant amount of blame for permitting this travesty to occur. Individually egotistical, envious of more successful colleagues and always willing participants in schemes that promise to enhance their personal influence, they are frequently too willing to follow the "yellow brick road".

Today, the medical profession lacks positive objectives and a united front, best characterized by inaction. The result, long waiting lists, diminishing quality of care; all consequences of collective passivity; Short-term thinking for permanent pain. One need only read the many popular novels in the marketplace today i.e. Michael Palmer's "Society", Michael Crichton's "State of Fear", etc. to fully comprehend the current state of affairs. Managed Health Care once hailed as the ideal model, equates to large profits for a few and misery for most.

Where does one go from here? Invariably, it is difficult to turn back the clock. Individuals must form cooperatives much on the same basis on which insurance companies were originally founded. These should be non-profit, whereby the individual controls his destiny, chooses his physician independently and on the basis of quality of care. Most importantly it removes the middle men of misery. Only by adapting this type of strategy can viable health care systems be ensured.

Social Commentary #3

Societal Culture and Health Care

In the age of nuclear fission and nanotechnology, the world is becoming a less gracious, gentle and tolerant place. Along with deteriorating, moral, educational and environmental standards, this trend is compounded by the exponentially growing stress factor. Additional negative influences include an expanding population concomitant with the depletion of the earth's essential resources, (i.e. water, energy, etc.). Combined with the expanding power and insatiable appetite for funds on the part of the bureaucracy and their political masters, existence is often intolerable or reduced to a struggle for survival.

P. B. Medawar, a noted British scientist, performed a number of experiments in the 1930's that clearly demonstrated things to come. In one of his experiments, frogs were placed in an environment where the heat was steadily increased a fraction of a degree on a daily basis. The frogs adapted to their environment until their protoplasm disintegrated. In another experiment using rats, it was demonstrated that an increase in population led to a level at which the animals developed hostile and destructive behavior, often resulting in cannibalization. These experiments reveal the adaptability of the organism and the point at which physical, mental and social breakdown occurs. Much as in Orwell's "1984" published over fifty years ago, society should take note.

Hans Selye, another leading scientist in the 1950's, began to focus on the influence of stress in our lives. He authored many books and articles pertaining to the negative aspects of this factor, which now increasingly dominates our lives. Many manifestations of this feature exist – the trials of air travel, inflation, rising energy prices, soaring taxes and the continuing accountability required by the numerous levels of government. All things begin at the top, therefore the unprincipled behavior that we witness in government at the highest level is mirrored by the conduct of large corporations, small business and individuals. As long as this trend is allowed to continue without serious effort to reverse it, our future remains dismal.

Personally, I abhor violence in any form, much as most civilized people do; moreover, I subscribe to the philosophy that it is never justifiable. In instances where the individual is the victim of selective persecution, the imposition of injustice particularly in the case of the vulnerable and poor, one must begin to weigh the problem versus the solution. Presently, the average citizen cannot afford the luxury of appropriate judicial representation. The axiom of "not guilty until proven otherwise," no longer exists. The principle of government "for the people by the people" has become a myth. Indeed, we have become the servants of government, accountable for all our actions, assets and activities, that is clearly an invasion of our individuality and privacy. Whereas I am not a fan of Martha Stewart, I feel that her costly prosecution and conviction were carried out on a selective basis, with the determination to prove her guilty regardless of all other considerations and whatever crime she may have committed. Without sounding cynical, the act she allegedly committed is repeated countless times in the securities industry on a daily basis.

At this point, one might ask what provokes relatively normal and even outstanding citizens to resort to sudden violence. Is it injustice perceived, justice denied or the inability to purchase the level of judicial expertise required to exonerate? The multiple recent episodes of violence directed towards judges, teachers and other members of the authoritarian class need to be evaluated at the causative level and appropriate measures to correct these problems must be initiated. Society and its leaders should review the reasons for these increasing aberrations, instead of sensationalizing the outcomes.

Clearly citizens belabored by the above pressures, just like the rats in Medawar's experiments can reach a breaking point. The mindless influence of the entertainment industry with its unrelenting violence and pornographic exploitation also sends the wrong message. These influences can only lead to more inappropriate actions rather than presenting solutions.

In Canada, similar to most countries around the globe, government directives are increasingly based on political considerations and expedience, rather than reality. Political energies and funds are expended on the electoral process and the subsequent consolidation of power in order to become re-elected. Inevitably, these maneuvers exhaust the energy required to govern. To fund these self-serving activities bureaucracies resort to further oppression by imposing an inequitable and expanding tax base, including the promotion of gambling, once prosecuted as a criminal activity by the same leaders.

The electorate in order to gain the attention of officialdom in its many forms should perhaps consider not endorsing current regimes until reform of the broadest measure can be initiated. This would include abstaining from the current voting process and withholding the payment of taxes, stimuli required to bring about the cessation of government malfeasance enacted on an accepted ongoing basis. Subsequently a meritocracy composed of individuals elected on the basis of ability should emerge.

In the age of technology, current forms of government have become obsolete no matter what terminology is in vogue. High-level professionals must be elected to implement laws that are just and based on the realities of the day, not on questionable polls. Should the electorate fail to address these problems we are relegated to continuing mediocrity and the inevitable collapse of our society.

Social Commentary #4

SOCIAL COMMENTARY
-The Insurance Industry and Medicine

The purpose of this article is to focus on the expanding role of insurance companies in the practice of medicine. Originally, insurance was instituted as a method to provide coverage for inordinate expenses. Over the past thirty years, this has progressed to the point where insurance corporations have assumed a large measure of control of the operation of the healthcare system. It begins with the insidious forms required to be completed by both patients and physicians in order to obtain coverage. These are labor intensive, intrusive and often beyond reason. As a busy physician, dealing with patients suffering from a variety of pathologies, I am motivated at this time to reflect on this undesirable state of affairs.

Once upon a time, patients came to the physician or other healthcare provider because they were ill. Routinely, a thorough physical examination was carried out to establish a diagnosis and subsequently appropriate treatment was instituted. This scenario has changed dramatically. Currently, when a patient presents in the consulting room and is asked the conventional question "What is your complaint?" – all too often they respond by stating, "the insurance company;" thereupon recounting a litany of the problems they encounter in their efforts to obtain payment. Whether a work related problem, an episode of trauma or other illness, the company has denied their claim even though they may have religiously paid premiums for over twenty years. At this point the battle begins. The variety of stories are endless and illustrate the many creative ways that insurance companies have developed to avoid discharging their obligations. As the tale unfolds, I continue with my paper work, allowing the patient to vent until exhausted. I then inform them, that although sympathetic to their cause, that the secretarial staff is trained to deal with this aspect of the situation. At the same time, I assure them that I will do whatever I can to assist with the resolution of this injustice.

Unfortunately, many patients today even when treatment is urgent, elect to lie in bed at home wallowing in self-pity until they can resolve the issue of "who pays for what." Some patients wisely decide to pay for their care independently and proceed to get well while others continue to wait until the insurance issue is resolved – which may be never. Clearly, there is something wrong with this equation, or am I the only member of the medial profession to be cognizant of this situation?

Frequently it would appear that it is the intent of the insurance company to stall for time - hoping the patient will disappear. The adage is that time overcomes all things. There is also the veiled intent to brand the patient as a malingerer or worse. Clearly, this type of activity is improper if not outright fraudulent on the part of the carrier. In the past, organizations have been established by insurers to resolve these disputes. Currently, they are known as DAC Centres. Unfortunately, these organizations are extremely biased in favor of the insurance carrier and anyone who believes that this process is equitable should have an IQ test along with a sanity assessment.

This brings to the fore the question, "Are insurance companies and adjusters qualified to make medical decisions and how did they obtain the license to do so - legitimately or by fiat?" Problems are further compounded that when the carrier does agree to authorize treatment they attempt to control all aspects of this process. Again is it the right of the companies' administrators to make a presumptive diagnosis and in essence determine the course of treatment. As a physician, I am forced to deal with this on a daily basis. I feel that it is necessary to question these intrusive and negative influences. More importantly, it must be determined, what can be done to rectify them?

When patients bring their problems to my attention, I suggest that they request a return of their premiums with compound interest for the period that they have paid to the insurance carrier. Sometimes this works and at other times it is necessary for them to resort to legal recourse in order to obtain satisfaction.

Eliot Spitzer, the attorney general of the state of New York, at this time is leading an intensive investigation of insurance carriers for conspiracy and price-fixing activities. Regardless of his motives, it is gratifying to see that this issue is being addressed.

Insurance companies are in the business of making large profits and do not really appear to be interested in providing coverage for patient's expenses, the original intent of the contract. For them premiums are fine - coverage is not. This is confirmed by banks already flush with profits currently taking over insurance companies, a process not designed to benefit patients. Whereas, this situation may not be universal it exists in a disturbing number of cases. Personally, I have neither the time nor funds to investigate this vexing problem, but strongly feel that formal investigations should be continued with appropriate answers and <u>resolutions</u> forthcoming.

About the Author

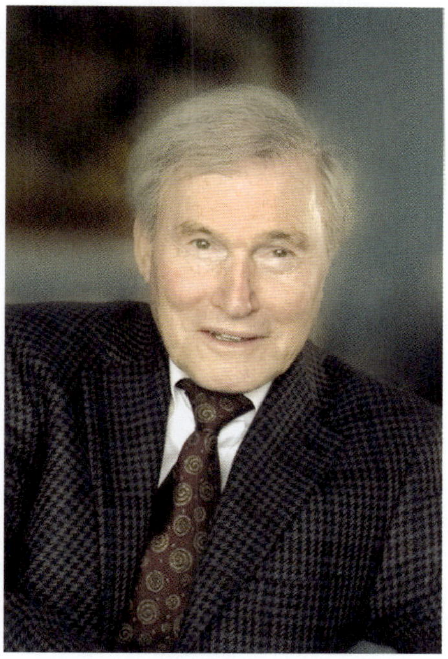

Fred Kahn, MD, FRCS(C)

Dr. Kahn is a graduate of the Faculty of Medicine at the University of Toronto. Following graduation, he initiated postgraduate studies to obtain his Fellowship of the Royal College of Surgeons of Canada and the Diplomate of the American Board of Surgery.

In 1988, Dr. Kahn discovered Low Intensity Laser Therapy and quickly grasped the significance of its healing potential. Accordingly, he combined the technical expertise of several engineering disciplines with the appropriate clinical objectives. This synergy gave birth to the most advanced Low Intensity Laser Therapy Unit globally, known as the 'BioFlex System". The process transformed a relatively primitive technology into the gold standard for the industry.

Dr. Kahn leads and teaches by example. The impact of his contribution to science may not have achieved the recognition it deserves today but will certianly do so in the future. In my opinion, eventually it will change the practice of medicine.

It is fortunate that he brought his profound energy and intellect to this task which benefits thousands of patients around the world on a daily basis. He has been and continues to be an inspiration to all who have worked with him and I speak for myself when I say, it has been a privilege to collaborate on this project.

Leslie C. Perrin

Leslie C. Perrin M.Sc., B.A. (Hon.)
Director of Laser Therapy Education
Certified Laser Therapist